The *Image* of *Nursing*

PERSPECTIVES ON SHAPING, EMPOWERING, AND ELEVATING THE NURSING PROFESSION

Shelley Cohen, RN, MS, CEN • Kathleen Bartholomew, RN, MN

HCPro

The Image of Nursing: Perspectives on Shaping, Empowering, and Elevating the Nursing Profession is published by HCPro, Inc.

ISBN:978-1-60146-247-3

HCPro, Inc., provides information resources for the healthcare industry.

HCPro, Inc., is not affiliated in any way with The Joint Commission, which owns the JCAHO and Joint Commission trademarks. MAGNET™, MAGNET RECOGNITION PROGRAM®, and ANCC MAGNET RECOGNITION® are trademarks of the American Nurses Credentialing Center (ANCC). The products and services of HCPro, Inc., and The Greeley Company are neither sponsored nor endorsed by the ANCC.

Photo Credit: RN patch is the product of an exhibition titled "RN: The Past, Present, and Future of the Nurse's Uniform." Mark Dion and J. Morgan Pruett in collaboration with the fabric workshop and Museum of Philadelphia. Used with permission. Nursing credential patches used with permission of the Center for Nursing Advocacy.

Shelley Cohen, RN, MS, CEN, Author
Kathleen Bartholomew, RN, MN, Author
Diana Swihart, PhD, DMin, MSN, CS, RN-BC, Contributing Author
Barbara J. Hannon, RN, MSN, CPHQ, Contributing Author
Karen L. Tomajan, MS, RN, BC, CNAA, CRRN, Contributing Author
Edie Brous, RN, MSN, MPH, JD, Contributing Author
Laura Cook Harrington, RN, MHA, CPHQ, CHCQM, Contributing Author
Rebecca Hendren, Associate Editorial Director
Patrick Campagnone, Cover Designer
Genevieve d'Entremont, Copyeditor
Sada Preisch, Proofreader
Jean St. Pierre, Senior Director of Operations

Advice given is general. Readers should consult professional counsel for specific legal, ethical, or clinical questions.

Arrangements can be made for quantity discounts. For more information, contact:

HCPro, Inc.
75 Sylvan Street, Suite A-101
Danvers, MA 01923
Telephone: 800/650-6787 or 781/639-1872
Fax: 781/639-2982
E-mail: *customerservice@hcpro.com*

Visit HCPro at
www.hcpro.com* and *www.hcmarketplace.com

Dedication

My image of nursing began to take shape back in 1965 as I walked to the J.B. Thomas Hospital in Peabody, MA, in my candy striper uniform. The image grew when I graduated from the Faulkner Hospital School of Nursing in 1975. Through all these phases, my parents were always proud of the icon I represented: the nurse. With this in mind, I dedicate this book to my mother, Marcia Cohen, and my late father, Albert Cohen.

As I work toward the future—pursuing another phase of image as I obtain my master's of nursing degree—it is my husband, Dennis, who beams with pride. His unconditional love and support provide me with the determination to mentor other nurses.

I am proud to share the pages of this book with all the nurses out there who are working hard to ensure that the image of nursing is our choice.

–Shelley Cohen, RN, MS, CEN

I would like to dedicate this book to my mentors: Professor Emeritus Genevieve M. Bartol, EdD, RN, CHN, and Professor Linda Westbrook, RN, PhD. For their constant guidance, encouragement, and support I am most deeply grateful.

–Kathleen Bartholomew, RN, MN

Table of Contents

Acknowledgments

Nursing credential patches featured in the cover art are provided courtesy of the Center for Nursing Advocacy. The initial "RN" patch was created by J. Morgan Puett and Mark Dion in association with their exhibit "RN: The Past, Present and Future of Nurses' Uniforms," which exhibited October 2003 – February 2004 at The Fabric Workshop and Museum in Philadelphia. The RN patch is used with permission from Ms. Puett and Mr. Dion.

The remaining patches were created by the Center for Nursing Advocacy with permission from Ms. Puett and Mr. Dion. The Center seeks to increase public understanding of the central, frontline role nurses play in modern healthcare. The focus of the Center is to promote more accurate, balanced, and frequent media portrayals of nurses and increase the media's use of nurses as expert sources. The Center's ultimate goal is to foster growth in the size and diversity of the nursing profession at a time of critical shortage; strengthen nursing practice, teaching and research; and improve the healthcare system.

For more information on the Center for Nursing Advocacy and to become involved in its campaigns, visit *www.nursingadvocacy.org*. The current work of Ms. Puett and Mr. Dion can be found at *www.mildredslane.com*.

Our thanks also go to Judy Leverette, RN, BSN, Narciss Cheatham, LPN-IV, Zilla Henrickson, RN, BSN, Christine Stearns, RN, BSN, and Reggie Smith, RN at Williamson Medical Center in Franklin, TN, for their help with this project and their commitment to the profession of nursing.

About the Authors

Shelley Cohen, RN, MS, CEN, is the founder and president of Health Resources Unlimited, a Tennessee-based healthcare education and consulting company (*www.hru.net*). Through her seminars for healthcare workers, Cohen provides tools and resources for delivering the best in patient care through coaching and educating. She frequently presents her work on leadership development and triage at national conferences and meetings.

When she is not speaking or teaching, Cohen works prn as a staff emergency department nurse and is working on her master's in nursing degree. She authors her monthly electronic publications—*Manager Tip of the Month* and *Triage Tip of the Month*—read by thousands of professionals across the United States.

She is an editorial advisor for *Strategies for Nurse Managers*, published by HCPro, Inc., and has been a frequent contributor to *Nursing Management* magazine. She is the author of *Critical Thinking in the Emergency Department: Skills to Assess, Analyze, and Act,* and the other books in the Critical Thinking series, and co-authored the book *A Practical Guide to Recruitment and Retention: Skills for Nurse Managers*, all published by HCPro, Inc.

With more than 30 years experience as a nurse, she continues to work as a staff nurse with past experiences at various levels of nursing leadership. Cohen also serves as executive director of a non-profit she founded with her husband Dennis (DoubleCreek), which is a retreat for children in foster care.

Kathleen Bartholomew, RN, MN, a registered nurse and counselor, uses the power of story from her experience as the manager of a large surgical unit to shed light on the challenges and issues facing nurses today. Her strength is her ability to link the academic world with the practical reality of the hospital. Her objective is to serve as a much-needed voice for nursing today.

Bartholomew has been a national speaker for the nursing profession for the past seven years. Recognizing that the culture of an institution is critical to patient safety, she speaks on building community in the workplace, improving nurse-physician relationships, and improving nurse-to-nurse relationships. *Speak Your Truth: Proven Strategies for Effective Nurse-Physician Communication* was published in 2004 as her master's thesis. She also wrote the bestselling *Ending Nurse-to-Nurse Hostility: Why Nurses Eat Their Young and Each Other* in 2006 and *Stressed Out About Communication Skills* in 2007, published by HCPro, Inc. Both her lectures and books reflect her passion and love of nursing.

About the Contributing Authors

Diana Swihart, PhD, DMin, MSN, CS, RN-BC, is a clinical nurse specialist in nursing education at the Bay Pines VA Healthcare System in Bay Pines, FL, and has a widely diverse background in many professional nursing arenas, theology, ministry, ancient Near Eastern studies, and archaeology. She is a member of the editorial advisory board for *Advance for Nurses,* Florida edition, and the advisory boards for *The Staff Educator* and *HCPro's Advisor to the ANCC Magnet Recognition Program®,* published by HCPro, Inc., and the Shared Governance Forum online. She is the author of *Shared Governance: A Practical Approach to Reshaping Professional Nursing Practice*, and the *Nurse Preceptor Training System*, both published by HCPro, Inc.

She has published and spoken on a number of topics related to nursing, shared governance, evidence-based practice, competency assessment, education, preceptorships, new employee orientation, servant leadership, workforce grants, and nursing professional development, both locally and nationally.

Swihart has served as an ANCC Magnet Recognition Program® appraiser and is currently an ANCC accreditation appraiser, the treasurer for the National Nursing Staff Development Organization, and adjunct faculty at South University and Trinity Theological Seminary and College of the Bible distance learning program. Her training and experiences, including those in academic and staff development education, give her a broad and balanced perspective of nursing that influences and colors all that she does as she creatively challenges and encourages others through professional nurse development in professional practice environments of care.

Laura Cook Harrington, RN, MHA, CPHQ, CHCQM, is the director of live events and continuing education and senior consultant at The Greeley Company, a division of HCPro, Inc. She is an experienced healthcare manager with extensive background in the areas of performance improvement, peer review, risk, case management, and credentialing. Harrington is a registered nurse, a certified professional in healthcare quality, and a fellow of the American Board of Quality Assurance & Utilization Review Physicians. Harrington graduated from Texas Woman's University with a bachelor's degree in nursing and a master's degree in healthcare administration.

Barbara J. Hannon, RN, MSN, CPHQ, has been the ANCC Magnet Recognition Program® (MRP) coordinator for the University of Iowa Hospitals & Clinic since 2002. As the coordinator, she wrote and edited the standards required by the MRP, organized and motivated the MRP champions from all the inpatient and outpatient units at University of Iowa Hospitals and Clinics; spearheaded MRP activities throughout the institution including fairs, contests, and potlucks to increase the visibility of the project; and headed a massive educational effort for the entire organization that included sessions for not only all the nurses, but physicians, administrators, and other clinical staff as well. Along with being coordinator, Hannon chairs the professional nursing practice committee and nursing retention committee and is involved in quality improvement activities for the department. She gives multiple talks and presentations on the MRP, shared governance, and evidence-based practice throughout the year.

Prior to being appointed the coordinator for UIHC, Hannon was an advanced practice nurse in nursing research and has been an ER nurse at the institution for 12 years. She holds a BSN and an MSN from the University of Iowa College of Nursing, and is active in ENA ENCARE program, and a member of Sigma Theta Tau.

Karen L. Tomajan, MS, RN, BC, CNAA, CRRN, is director, nursing quality and special projects at INTEGRIS Baptist Center, an ANCC Magnet Recognition Program® (MRP) recognized facility in Oklahoma City. In this capacity, she edited the MRP self study and led staff education in preparation for the site visit. Tomajan precepts graduate students in the Clinical Nurse Leader program at the University of Oklahoma College of Nursing and serves as a program evaluator for the NLNAC. She recently authored an online module on facilitating staff development in the evidence-based Nurse Manager Certificate Program for Sigma Theta Tau and is the current president of the Oklahoma Nurses Association. During her career, she has served in a number of roles including staff nurse, charge nurse, staff educator, recruiter, academic educator, and director of nursing in rehabilitation, medical-surgical, geriatric and critical care settings. She lectures on team training concepts, lean thinking, nurse retention, and workforce advocacy strategies.

Tomajan is a strong advocate for workforce advocacy—a model for addressing workplace issues espoused by the Center for American Nurses—and is passionate about the power nurses have to make a difference in their own practice and collectively change the work environment for nurses and the patients they serve.

Edie Brous, RN, MSN, MPH, JD, is a nurse attorney in private practice in New York City, where she specializes in professional licensure representation, medical malpractice defense, and nursing advocacy. She serves on the board of directors for The American Association of Nurse Attorneys and the Center for Nursing Advocacy. She has an extensive clinical and managerial background in operating room, emergency, and critical care nursing. She coordinates the Legal Clinic column in the *American Journal of Nursing* and serves as a peer reviewer for several professional nursing journals. She is a contributing chapter author on several textbooks and is currently coauthoring and editing a textbook on legal and ethical issues for advanced practice nurses.

Foreword

Today's nurses face tremendous challenges on every shift. Our work is more intense and more complex, yet we have less time to deliver nursing care due to the decreased length of time patients remain in the hospital. Nurses must constantly integrate new technological discoveries, while pharmacological advances have resulted in patients living longer with chronic illness, multiple admitting diagnoses, and more medications. Every day nurses feel the effect of America's dysfunctional healthcare system, which ultimately asks nursing to compensate for its excess waste by adding tasks or failing to provide adequate resources. Regulatory concerns that attempt to address quality and safety continue to ask nurses to do more with less. All this can make the future appear overwhelming.

But there is something you can do immediately that will forever have a powerful and sustained affect on the future of nursing. Our image is a collective expression of the pride and professionalism each nurse feels and then portrays to the other members of the healthcare team and to society. There is no healthcare without nursing care, and the time has come for you to define your value through actions, conversations, and ideas. We don't have to wait for increased budgets or massive healthcare changes. We can take ownership of our image right now.

It is our hope that this book will give you the awareness, support, information, and tools needed to advance your professional image. One nurse at a time, we can and will affect our collective image. Will you join and support a professional nursing organization, mentor the next generation of nurses, and uphold the highest level of professionalism in your words and actions? It's your choice, your image.

–Shelley Cohen and Kathleen Bartholomew

One Profession, Many Images: Where Has Florence Nightingale Gone?

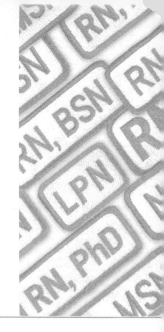

By Shelley Cohen, RN, MS, CEN

LEARNING OBJECTIVES

After reading this chapter, the participant will be able to:

✔ Discuss the current image of the nursing profession

✔ Recognize the effect of image on public perception

Formal Introductions

"This is my daughter, the nurse."

Some introduction from a parent, isn't it? But this is how I was always introduced: "the nurse" rather than my given name. Thinking back, I remember being bothered by this. At that time I felt my identity was more about who I was than what I was. But as I grew older I learned an important life lesson: Sometimes *what* you are really is *who* you are. Or at least it is when you are a nurse.

I have always been proud to be a nurse, and I have worked as a nurse with pride, beginning from the time I graduated to now, 33 years later, working as an educator and an emergency department staff nurse. Yet I find myself conflicted about the current image of nursing, and I feel something has changed. If my pride in being a nurse has not changed, then what has?

My feelings have changed due to many perspectives, and are in large part based on what I see in the nursing profession. I no longer see pride being demonstrated through what nurses wear, what they say, or how they act. I must add that this is a generalization and does not apply to every nurse. Many of us would never check a text message while talking to a patient or patient's family member. Many of us would not consider it an option to wear the same shoes to work that we wore while mowing the lawn that morning. Some of us might wonder what you were thinking if you suggested it was acceptable to place an online shopping order for a new pair of shoes while at work.

Through actions such as these and attitudes we hear about every day, one can conclude that many nurses do not take pride in their profession. What do you think when you hear nurses say, "I would never recommend my daughter go to nursing school—it's the most thankless job" or "We always get treated poorly; that's what it means to be a nurse these days."

Ouch. This hurts both to type and to read. How do you feel each time you hear the phrase "Nurses eat their young"? Doesn't that just make you feel special—only in the wrong way?

The perspectives on nursing image discussed in this text are not meant to serve as a journey down memory lane simply as a way for us to say, "Back in my early days of nursing you would never . . . " Statements like that are hogwash! Nursing has had trouble with its image for decades—it just didn't feature so much technology or shoes that had holes in them. Take nurse-to-nurse hostility as just one example: I can still feel a chill in my spine from the intimidation attempts thrown at me in 1975 when I first started work.

Many of us in the profession are starting to seriously examine our image and all its ramifications. If appearance, actions, and thoughts don't bring you to a place where you question the image of a nurse, try this one: How do you feel when the phrase "he or she is such a good nurse" is used to describe a nurse who has good clinical skills but also has a negative attitude and will not work with the team? Shouldn't being a good nurse imply one has skill *and* character? Are we saying that the minimum we will accept for a good nurse is skill?

Are other qualifiers no longer necessary to define a good nurse? Caring for patients as a team effort, encouraging one another, and supporting new graduates as they transition from student to professional are still important qualities for a nurse. Aren't they?

Writing About Image

By 2006, I found myself increasingly confronted with comments and personal experiences related to perceptions of nursing pride, nursing image, and what makes up a good nurse. I was on overload and needed to put my thoughts down on paper to release my pressure valve of frustration. Balancing somewhere between disappointment and concern over what had become of nursing and its image, I felt it was time to find some balance in all of this. With few resources available then, I gathered a sampling of data from a survey of more than 300 emergency department nurses related to their perceptions of their image. These results were presented at the Emergency Nurse Association 2007 Leadership Conference in Boston. Unsure as to what type of response I would get from the participants, I approached the presentation through the title *Perception Is Reality: The Image of the ED Nurse*. The feedback I received from this presentation was the affirmation I needed: I am not alone in my quest for the pride and image of nursing.

Others have also published recently on issues of image and perception. In the article "Nursing: Today and Beyond," Cindy Saver, RN, MS, (2006) took us on a journey that examined trends in nursing, and compared nursing by generation, from the days of ironing your nurses' cap and not wearing gloves to start an IV. Spurred by this article and others, the timing was perfect to once again raise some questions and continue my search for nursing pride, professionalism, and image. *American Nurse Today* published an article I wrote on "The Image of Nursing" as a cover piece in the May 2007 issue. This article caused quite a stir, and the editors of the journal told me they received more feedback than they ever expected. Nurses were starting to ask questions about image and pride, and they did this in letters to the editors and direct e-mails to me.

At this point, I recognized it was time to gather perspectives from educators, staff nurses, new graduates, and others in the field of nursing, and examine the issue from a wider perspective. In 2008, I took elements from the 2006 survey for ED nurses and reformatted it for nurses across all specialties and sent it out to nurses across the country. I received more than 1,000 responses to the survey, and I heard from others who have also been searching for the impact and impression of nursing. You may be tempted to fast-forward your reading to Chapter 2 to view these results; go ahead if you must. However, I encourage each reader to make time to listen and truly hear the perspectives of each contributing author. Chapter 11 will require you to take action as well as stimulate you to ask yourself some questions.

Historical Perspective

Think about all the descriptive names that have been applied to nursing throughout the years. Just the thought of some of these descriptors and stereotypes will give us enough debate to last a lifetime. From angels of mercy to handmaidens or glorified waitresses, for many, one name says it all.

But it's time to ask, who elected themselves in charge of deciding what our image should be?

Perhaps the more important question is, "Who took over the decision about our image while nursing was arguing amongst itself?" Did any of us anticipate that it would be the catalogue companies selling scrub uniforms who would dictate the visual image of a nurse? One quick glance at any catalogue will show you pages and pages of scrubs decorated with cartoon characters.

Think back to when nurses would:

- Rise to give their seat to a physician

- Tolerate a physician throwing an instrument at them as "part of the job"

- Smoke at the nurses' station

- Never think of wearing anything other than a white uniform (with a blue cardigan if they needed warmth)

Stay with me on this retro journey, and you may even recall a series of books featuring a nurse called Cherry Ames (which, by the way, is making a comeback). Any young girl with hopes of being a nurse in the early 1950s through the late 1960s was awestruck at everything this fictional character accomplished.

If you want to return to the birth of nursing, we are all drawn to Florence Nightingale, whose vision was beyond her time. A remarkable woman, her *Notes on Nursing* continue to amaze us more than 100 years later. The Florence Nightingale Museum Web site reminds us that her greatest achievement was *"to raise nursing to the level of a respectable profession for women"* (*www.florence-nightingale.co.uk*). She had in her mind what the image of nursing needed to be back then, and I believe that we forgot to continue to care for it in her absence.

The public perception of nursing is not accurate, and there is a distinct lack of realistic role models on television. In Chapter 3, author Karen Tomajan will walk you through her perceptions of the media's effect on our image and what is being done about it.

Defining Nursing's Image

Have we defined what nursing's image is, or do we first need to define what it is not? Results of our survey tell us what affects our image, but do we understand what comprises that image? Multitudes of resources list a variety of words to define "image," with the following being the most frequently cited:

- Reflection

- Idea

- Concept

- Representation

Using these four nouns, how would you define our image? How do you think your coworkers and family or friends would define it? What do they look for or listen to when responding? Do their responses come from personal experience or the television news? Is our image part of professionalism?

Our image is composed of many components that specify something about nursing as a healthcare profession. Our skill, education, what we say, how we act on and off duty, what we wear, and what we communicate about ourselves all paint a picture that creates this image. For example, our

survey revealed that 87.7% of nurses (781 in the sample) felt that whether or not we introduce ourselves as nurses has a great effect on our image. I wonder how patients would respond to this question and how it affects their perception of nursing each time they have to ask us the question, "Are you my nurse?" What perception is left when nurses do not introduce themselves as the nurse? Have you ever known a police officer to walk up to an individual and say, "I'm Mr. Jones" or "I'm Ken Jones"? They will introduce themselves as "Officer Jones" or say, "I am Sergeant Jones."

The best of intentions may be misperceived by coworkers, patients, and their families. The least-skilled nurse stepping into the exam room of Mrs. Bartlett, a 24-year-old obstetric patient, may be perceived as "wonderful" by this patient. You may hear things that relay messages of "how wonderful my nurse was today." What was it about this nurse that imparted this "wonderful" image? Was it something he/she was wearing that a 24-year-old connected with? Was it something he/she said or how he/she acted? The best-skilled nurse can approach a family member in crisis while a loved one is being cared for and leave an impression of fear and distrust. How can this happen with a skilled nurse? Was it something she wore, said, or did or did not do?

Image is affected by many considerations, but the considerations just discussed have to do with actions, clothing, introductions, etc. As we look for answers to the question of who is shaping the image of the nursing profession, we must look at healthcare roles that affect our image and its perception. For just a moment, slip on the shoes of a new graduate nurse. For some of you, no matter how far back this takes you, you can still recall the emotions, concerns, and fears of making the transition to staff nurse. For some, the wounds are still fresh, while others are glowing from the overt support and guidance they were showered with at their first nursing job. Who are the individuals who affected these new graduate nurses and what roles did they play?

Walk alongside a nurse traveler who is taking a position to help a medical-surgical floor meet its patient care caseload in the face of a nursing shortage. There are no welcome signs here, just some directions to the bathroom and the coffee pot if he or she is lucky. Instead of being welcoming and grateful for the help of another nurse, the nurses on this unit are aloof and do not display an image of professionalism. What persons played a part in this display, and what made them think this was acceptable behavior as a professional?

It starts at the top

As with many things in healthcare, what happens at the top is a reflection of how things are at the patient care level. When nurse leaders or managers arrive for work looking like they just rolled out of bed, why should staff think their appearance is important? You can have all the dress codes you want, but if leadership is not complying or holding others accountable, the impact is in the reflection. This also holds true for other elements related to image and professionalism. We need our nurse leaders to role-model the image, to set the tone, to walk and talk what is acceptable.

When you hear a nurse leader use foul language at a staff meeting or verbally berate the Board of Nursing for a standard, we have a problem "We" is the staff, patients and their families, and the rest of the healthcare team. A nurse manager I have worked with not only ensures she has a clean set of neat scrubs in her office should the need arise, she holds all staff accountable. If your name is on your

nursing license, then this manager expects you to comply with your state practice act as well as to demonstrate yourself as a professional. Another nurse manager I know violates organizational smoking policies, does not meet the dress code requirements, and when new staff reveal less than professional interactions, they are told to "get over it." Like it or not, the reality is that we have a wide variability amongst our nurse leaders and their image. You have a very short period of time for staff to figure out who you are; first impressions always have and always will make a difference.

Appearance shapes perception

Let me share an example of a time I worked with an organization and I had an interaction with their clinical specialist nurse. What type of image would you expect when you hear "clinical nurse specialist"? Have you started to visualize how he or she might look? Imagine a clinical specialist introducing him or herself to a patient he or she is consulting on. What type of image do you think the patient is visualizing? Well, take a pin to that bubble, because what I was confronted with was a disheveled nurse, wearing an outfit you might wear to pick up groceries or the newspaper. Did I mention the clinical specialist was text messaging while we talked?

Is this the image we want a master's-level nurse to portray? It does not matter how many degrees she had or years of experience. Your confidence in this person is instantly affected by the image she reflects. What made her think this is an acceptable appearance for a clinical specialist to have? Do we really need to put in writing for every level of nurse that they must show up to work looking professional?

The image of nursing is affected when interactions occur between healthcare workers, both in front of the patient and behind closed doors. Kathleen Bartholomew addresses these head on in Chapter 6. What happens when you see unacceptable behaviors from another nurse or healthcare worker? For many of you the answer is "nothing"; the response is, "They always act like that." And that makes it okay?

A nurse preceptor who assisted with orientation of new hires and new graduates was also involved in some classroom activities the department held. She always showed up looking neat and professional, never in blue jeans. When other staff would challenge her with "What are you so dressed up for?" she would respond with a very important message about image. She would share with staff that to ensure new hires took the classroom experience seriously, it was important she seemed professional, not just in her presentation but in her appearance as well.

What image is left behind when a family member approaches the clinic nurse to ask a question about the patient only to find the nurse face-down engrossed in text messaging? What concept is delivered when a nurse delegates nonnursing functions to unlicensed staff? What perception is left in the minds of those who witness the charge nurse verbally berating another nurse? When was the last time you had a physician recognize you and your worth as a professional nurse? This past year I had a physician approach me to thank for me being there and reminded me how important I was to the department. Someone please pinch me because I think I am dreaming!

What a wonderful experience to have that recognition from a provider. The more I thought about it, the more I realized this should not be a rare occurrence. Looking back, I wish I had asked him what prompted the comment.

One nurse follows another's work, day after day and shift after shift. Whether it is in the office/clinic, home health, school, or inpatient setting, you are starting with the leftovers from the previous nurse. How many times has a patient or family member said any of the following?

- Where is Tim today? I miss seeing him. He is such a great nurse.

- I am so glad to see you today. Finally, a nurse who actually cares.

- I hate to say anything to anyone, but that other nurse . . .

- I didn't know he/she was a nurse. I could have asked him/her, but he/she never said anything about being the nurse.

- I wish all the nurses were as nice as you are.

- I didn't know nurses could do that.

- I hate to ask the doctor this question, but I know I can ask you because you're a nurse.

Being in the position of hearing some of these comments can be quite uncomfortable, while other comments bring confirmation of professionalism and a job well done.

Shaping the image of nursing requires actions on the part of all healthcare workers, but it has to start with the nurse first. I continuously hear from nurses that our profession is not respected by others. Why should it be? Sandy Dumont, an image consultant, who has directed the image of executives for more than 25 years, states, "You're the only thing between patients and death, and you're covered in cartoons" (Raymond 2004). Have you ever seen a police officer or firefighter or paramedic with Snoopy stickers all over his or her uniform? What other profession has allowed uniform catalogue companies to decide what their visual image should be? Cute doesn't help the frightened parent of a child who is critically ill. What you perceive as appearing "fun" or appealing to the patient/family you care for may leave a very different impression with those on the viewing side. One comment from a patient who happened to like your uniform does not constitute a research project. One of my staff positions required purchasing solid black scrubs for uniforms. My thoughts? *How much more morbid can you get?* But feedback from the viewer's side included:

- You look so professional

- I like your outfit—it looks like you got dressed up for me

- Everyone here looks so nice

Many nurses feel that certain patient popula-tions, such as hospice patients and pediatric patients, respond better when the nurse is dressed differently. I believe this is true for certain situations, but can people tell who is the nurse? Can you visually be differentiated from ancillary services such as lab and housekeeping? I have worked with pediatric patients for more than 30 years and never had a problem relating to them without cartoons on my uniform. Blowing bubbles, a gentle voice and touch, a stuffed animal, and a little humor go a long way no matter what your uniform is.

It's important to remember we are great at what we do no matter what we are wearing. The point is that the perception of our abilities and competencies from the patient/family perspective is based partly on our appearance. Our survey results revealed that 90.6 % (819) nurses felt that how they dress had a great impact on their image. One respondent wrote, "I would insist on having a national nursing white professional uniform." While wearing white is an issue that many disagree with, what is wrong with having one national professional uniform, so we can be recognized as nurses? With recognition comes respect. Take your image back—your reflection is in the mirror.

How Individuals Can Shape Our Image

The national image survey asked respondents what individual nurses can do to help Shape a more realistic image of nursing. Following are some of the surprising and not- so-surprising remarks. (You can view all of the responses at: *www.strategiesfornursemanagers.com*).

Adopt more professional behaviors at the nurse's station, with the patient, and in the community.

Appear as an educated professional. I believe so many nurses make themselves out to be catty, high school type women/men, and this greatly affects how others view our profession. Look, act, behave as a professional.

Remember that a professional nurse always projects a professional image, even when the circumstances she/he finds self in are trying. This is true even when (perhaps especially when) you are not being treated as, or recognized as a professional.

By always having a caring attitude but professional. We are spread very thin but it does not help to "whine" to patients.

Dress and act more professionally. I know nurses are under a lot of stress trying to meet the needs of families, the patients, the doctors, and administrators, but we need not "make a scene or get an attitude."

By remembering that people are always watching and judging everything you do as a nurse. Your behavior at work and in the community should always be professional.

The professionalism standard needs to be reinforced. Nurses need to understand the full meaning of professionalism.

Be a professional. Be proactive. Stop laziness among nurses. It is your job whether you like it or not. Change careers if you don't like it.

Be nice. Stop backstabbing and sabotaging each other at work. Think best of each other. However, be willing to step up and address these negative behaviors with each other.

Have respect for themselves and others. Don't put your career in a box and forget about it. Don't limit what you do by being only task oriented. Go outside of your comfort zone. Grow and share what you know you know. Don't let patients think what a non-nursing coworker thinks of nurses: "They came into my room but didn't do anything except take my blood pressure." "They gave me my medicine but really didn't know what they were doing." "I had so many of them and couldn't remember

NURSING VOICES

any of them doing anything to help me get well." "I think I'd rather have a good doctor instead of a good nurse."

Introduce ourselves to patients as a Registered Nurse, discuss our body of scientific knowledge in the public; stop saying that "we work too hard" and speak of the honor involved in our profession.

Have a Bachelor's Degree and a Master's Degree. We require it of our teachers, why not our nurses?

Dress and act professionally. Be genuine with her patients & their families. Caring attitude. Keep informed on changes & show confidence to your patient that you know what you are doing.

Accountability for your actions and practice.

Be professional, we have lost that.

Be aware of your "audience." Older folks do not like Sponge Bob and psychedelic tops. If you do wear brighter scrubs be sure they are clean and neat, not with buttons falling off and pockets drooping. And pay attention to your shoes!! I wear crocs myself, but they go through the wash weekly and don't look like they were stolen from the local garbage heap.

Stay updated. Act professional. Demand excellence from others as well as ourselves.

Sell what we do in a realistic but positive light. Promote the impact of even the smallest moments of caring—it is not all about the biggest arrests, the goriest traumas or those bloody TV shows! Individual nurses need to tell their stories more, they are incredibly powerful. Nurses need to stand for what is nursing, and not let it be devalued by skill replacement with cheaper labor. Nurse leaders need to lead this, instead of supporting nurse replacement with less qualified nurses as 'the answer' to the aging nursing workforce. Individual nurses need to be striving for, permitting, and encouraging true workforce flexibility in shift patterns, hours of work, and the ability to be promoted on the basis of true ability to do the job best, not on being able to work the 'establishment hours'.

Bring back professionalism—we seem to have lost it. Nurses need to treat each other and colleagues and other healthcare workers with respect. Treat each other as team members, in which we all play a part in caring for patients, no one is more important than others we just function in different roles.

REFERENCES

Cohen, S. (2007). "The image of nursing: How do others see us? How do we see ourselves?" *American Nurse Today* 2 (5): 24-26.

Florence Nightingale Museum. (2008). Available at *www.florence-nightingale.co.uk*.

Nightingale, F. (1859). *Notes on Nursing: What It Is, and What It Is Not.* London, England: Harrison and Sons, Bookseller to the Queen.

Raymond, P. (2004). "Nursing image = Nursing power." Available at *www.theimagearchitect.com*.

Saver, C. (2006). "Nursing: Today and Beyond." *American Nurse Today* 1 (1):18-25.

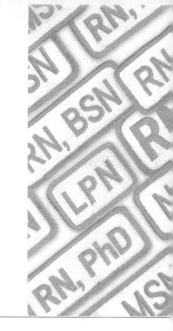

CHAPTER 2

Survey Says: Results from National Nursing Image Survey

By Shelley Cohen, RN, MS, CEN

After reading this chapter, the participant will be able to:

✔ Discuss the results of a national nursing survey regarding image

Hearing from Our Peers

In preparation for this book, I felt it was essential to ask nurses around the country about their thoughts on our image and whether they had concerns, and I decided to use a survey as the method for feedback. The survey was active from the months of April 2008 through June 2008, and feedback was requested through an online survey program.

One thousand one hundred and forty-two nurses responded to the survey and gave their opinions and perceptions about the image of the nursing profession. To protect the privacy of the participants, they did not have to disclose any contact information in order to enter their responses. Questions for the survey were selected with the following considerations:

- Keep the survey short to encourage participants to complete all questions

- Use pointed questions about issues that directly affect image and professionalism

- Provide at least one entry area for narrative opinion of the participant

Survey results for questions one through seven were analyzed through the survey Web site's programming. I reviewed and categorized the narrative responses for questions eight and nine. This self-administered approach fit the timeline of the preparation of the book and made it more user-friendly to those interested in responding. The purpose of this survey was to initiate a forum that would produce substantial data about how nurses perceive their image and what they believe directly affects it. As with many surveys, there are certain limitations, and this one was no different. You will note as you review the results that only 1% of the responses are from new graduate nurses and 70% are from nurses with more than 15 years of experience.

To ensure more perspectives from the student nurse and new graduate nurse, you will note comments and opinions from their perspective distributed in various elements of this book. It is essential for the profession to make a connection across the entire continuum of the profession: from student, to novice, to experienced nurse.

It would have been of interest to also note perceptual differences between staff nurses and nurse leaders. Several additional questions were considered for this survey, such as specialty, position, and years at current position, among others. I recommend that these results serve as a springboard for an expanded survey that can be applied as evidence for changes in practice.

SURVEY RESULTS

Question 1. Gender

Male	Female
8.3%	91.7%

Question 2. Age

<30	31–50	51–60	>60
6.1%	51.2%	37.5%	5.2%

Question 3. Years experience as a nurse

New graduate	<3	3–5	6–9	10–15	>15
1%	4%	5.2%	5.2%	14.6%	70%

Question 4. Location

United States	Other country
97.7%	2.3%

 The Image of Nursing

SURVEY RESULTS

Question 5. Rate the following as to your opinion on how each item affects the image of the nurse

	Has NO effect on image	Has LITTLE effect on image	Has GREAT effect on image	Response count
How we present ourselves to patient/family	0.2% (2)	0.9% (9)	**98.9% (1,031)**	**1,042**
How we dress	0.3% (3)	9.4% (98)	**90.3% (938)**	**1,039**
How skilled we appear to be at our jobs	0.3% (3)	3.5% (36)	**96.3% (1,003)**	**1,042**
Misinformation from TV and other media	0.4% (4)	21.8% (226)	**77.8% (808)**	**1,038**
Whether or not we introduce ourselves as nurse	0.5% (5)	12.0% (125)	**87.5% (912)**	**1,042**
How we appear to get along with coworkers	0.5% (5)	12.8% (133)	**86.7% (899)**	**1,037**
Whether or not we belong to a professional nursing organization	22.0% (229)	**54.3% (565)**	23.7% (246)	**1,040**
How we act around nurses' station, etc.	0.1% (1)	5.3% (55)	**94.6% (981)**	**1,037**
Whether or not patient/family feels we care	0.2% (2)	1.2% (12)	**98.6% (1,023)**	**1,037**
How easily patient/family can read our name tags	2.1% (22)	43.5% (451)	**54.4% (564)**	**1,037**
Answered question				1,042
Skipped question				118

SURVEY RESULTS

Question 6. Do you feel disruptive behaviors among and between staff nurses (horizontal violence) has affected our image?

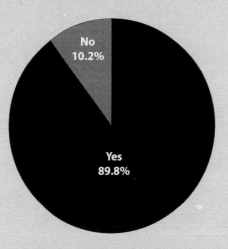

Question 7. Do you think having a Bachelor's Degree in nursing impacts the image a nurse has?

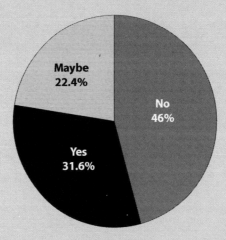

SURVEY RESULTS

Question 8. What do you think the individual nurse can do to help shape a more realistic image of nursing?

807 participants responded to this question, with 353 skipping it.

For ease of reviewing, I elected to group responses to questions 8 and 9 into categories. The following six categories reflected the theme of the responses:

❖ *Appearance*

Responses that fell into this category included strong messages of discontent with not only dress code concerns, but also what we appear to be doing at work, such as eating at the nurses' station. Comments included:

- Wear your ID badge

- Stop the cartoon scrubs

- Don't dress like a slob

- We are professional, so we must act like it

- Be aware of your audience; older folks do not like Sponge Bob and psychedelic tops

- When nurses end their shift and go to a bar in scrubs, it cheapens our image

❖ *Behavior*

Responses that fell into this category related to acting professionally and not complaining in public about our job. Backstabbing and sabotage were frequently noted as concerns, as was the need to work together as a team. Many expressed a desire for nurses to talk positively about the profession in public, along with being kind, helpful, and compassionate. Comments included:

- If you don't like the profession—get out.

- We are always onstage, even at the ballpark—talk positively about the profession.

- Realize that nursing is a career, not just a job. We are professional so we must act like it.

- Be nice and stop backstabbing each other at work.

- Nurses that bad-mouth the profession should be encouraged to leave the profession.

- Promote a professional image; act professional.

- Be respectful to everyone.

SURVEY RESULTS

– Stop the bickering and do your job.

– There is a familiar phrase that has always haunted me, "Nurses eat their young." And boy do they— nurses are the unfriendliest group of people I have ever been around.

❖ *Communication skills*

Responses in this category expressed a need for the profession to be a positive voice and called for nurses to speak up for themselves more often. Respondents identified a need for nurses to learn more effective communication skills and to introduce themselves to their patients as the nurse. Their suggestions included:

– Smile; speak in a clear, pleasant voice

– Use eye contact, be empathetic

– We can communicate what we find in assessments to the patient as well as the MD; people think we change beds—they have no clue what the RN does

– Communicate with our patients

– Speak intelligently all the time

– Speak to patients and families in a caring manner

❖ *Education/competency*

Much discussion here related to encouraging other nurses to achieve specialty certification and continue ongoing education. Some discussion related to setting the BSN education level as the minimum entry into nursing. Suggestions included:

– One type of entry-level requirements that are consistent across the board.

– Always look for ways to learn.

– Demonstrate competency.

– Keep up with clinical research updates and be objectively open-minded.

– Current entry-level nursing is the most uneducated in the healthcare field. Shame on us.

– Insist on three months of orientation for new grads.

– Take greater ownership accountability—obtain specialty certification.

SURVEY RESULTS

❖ Professional organizations

Strength in numbers was the theme noted in this category, with respondents suggesting that we can improve our image with more involvement in nursing organizations. Twenty-three point seven percent of the responses to this survey indicated that belonging to a professional nursing organization would have a great impact on our image. Specific comments related to this included:

- We are the largest of healthcare groups in the U.S. and it seems as if we have limited control of the issues affecting healthcare.

- Belong to nursing organizations—then an individual's voice will be combined with others to make positive changes—together we can achieve a lot.

- We have no one who represents nursing. As individuals we have no power.

- Be involved in professional nursing organizations and make yourself visible to the public.

❖ Public education/awareness

Many respondents felt that nursing has not done a good job of educating the public on nursing's various roles. A theme of being more proactive in our communities emerged, with recommendations for more involvement and better utilization of opportunities to improve awareness of the profession. These thoughts included:

- Offer to be a source for local and state politicians

- Be proactive in the community—when people can put an "everyday" face to the profession, it really helps to shape people's opinions, both good and bad

- Educate the public on what we do

- Advocate for ourselves; put forth a more united front

- Represent nursing at schools and scouts and other functions, so the upcoming generation has an accurate picture

- Make time to help "quantify" what nurses do in studies, etc.

- Educate family, friends, and public that the role of the nurse today requires extensive knowledge, critical thinking, astute judgment, and advanced decision-making skills in addition to empathy and compassion. Campaign against the media for poor portrayals of nurses, e.g., the TV show *Scrubs*.

SURVEY RESULTS

Question 9. If you had the power to change ONE thing about nursing that you feel would have the greatest impact on our image, what would that one thing be?

821 participants responded to this question, with 339 skipping it.

❖ *Education requirements for nursing*

As we saw in the responses to question 8, concern regarding the lack of a standard entry requirement in the nursing profession was evident. Requiring a BSN was the most common recommended minimum level of education.

- Four-year degree as basic entry; grandfather in those that do not have a degree. Time to stop arguing and move forward toward a professional practice.

- Require a professional education.

- Universal education preparation.

- BSN would help to demonstrate that nurses are professionals.

- No other profession has a double standard for minimum education requirements.

- Get rid of the two-year RN programs.

- Baseline for entry into virtually every other educated profession is a bachelor's degree.

❖ *Unity*

Unifying the profession through unions and active engagement in local and national activities was a strong message. Many noted that we could find strength in our numbers.

- Becoming a cohesive political unit

- Unionization

- Unite the profession

- Unionize all nurses across the USA into one big union . . . strength in numbers

- To have nurses gather together and project one voice

- Have a major walkout so the public, doctors, and admin could appreciate what we actually do

- I would like us to all stick together

SURVEY RESULTS

- Our professional organizations should not be unions in disguise

- Have a united front . . . Nurses are our own worst enemy

❖ *Appearance*

How we look and present ourselves was discussed from many perspectives. The reality of how we appear versus how the media portrays nurses was a concern in these responses.

- For nurses not to be viewed as sex symbols.

- Uniforms.

- Return to a professional image of a nurse. White uniforms and nursing caps.

- More men in managerial positions.

- I would insist on having a national nursing white professional uniform.

- Get rid of the TV/media images.

- I would make a mandatory dress code for nurses in both acute care and long-term care.

❖ *Staffing concerns*

Nurses who responded felt that we are perceived as always being in a rush, with little time to spend with the patient and families. They felt that this perception affects how others see us as professionals. Concerns about staffing levels were identified as an obstacle to our ability to provide many of the professional aspects of nursing care.

- Better staffing ratios

- The more staff you have, the better service you can provide

- Do something about the shortage so that nurses have time to care for each patient

- Mandate less patient load . . . which could improve nurses' attitudes/lessen stress levels and would allow patients to feel as if they are receiving better nursing care

- Nurses are burning out

- I can honestly say that adequate staffing would encourage a more caring attitude

SURVEY RESULTS

❖ *Behavior*

The focus here was a need for more respect amongst nurses, as well as with other healthcare workers with whom we collaborate. Frequently mentioned was the relationship between nursing and medicine.

- Nurses' attitudes

- How the older generation is disrespectful to the younger generation

- Stop the bickering and backstabbing

- A few bad apples spoil the whole bunch

- That it is a predominately female profession

- Our constant complaints—we really need to be positive and stop the never-ending conversations of complaints

- That we be treated as colleagues and peers of the physicians

- Provide each nurse with the ability to communicate the needs of the profession in a productive manner

- How we present ourselves at the bedside

- For nurses in general, to quit bad-mouthing the profession

- Treat each other with respect

You can view the full narrative entries for questions 8 and 9 in the benchmarking report section of *www.StrategiesForNurseManagers.com*, an online resource for nurse managers.

When you evaluate the responses and compare them to your personal perceptions, you will find some you agree with and others you disagree with. This is about finding a common ground that most nurses can agree on regarding how we can effect changes that positively impact our image. Take the time to visit *www.strategiesfornursemanagers.com* and review more responses. You might be surprised at the answers.

An important step in critiquing responses to a survey is to look at the strength and validity of the responses and their applicability to the question or problem raised. As we explore some of the history and rationale behind the themes identified, our hope is to provide the reader with a better understanding of how the image we own today as nurses evolved. From there, it is up to us to work together as a unified profession and decide the image of the nurse for tomorrow. While surveys, research, and journal articles provide a wealth of information about image, we can also gain much from listening to a personal perspective.

All voices need to be heard in order for nursing to present a unified image. In the Personal Perspective that follows, nursing student Jenna Sanders shares her perspective. As you read about her experiences, you can feel good that the future of nursing is being left in the hands of nursing students such as Jenna. You make us proud Jenna!

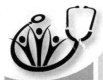

Personal Perspectives: Current Nursing Student

By Jenna Sanders

It was fall of 2003, and I had just given birth to my third child. My first two children were four and three years old, and I had what by all standards was the ideal life. My husband, a computer software consultant, supported the family quite well, and I had been able to stay at home with my children for the last three years. I was reasonably certain, up until that point, that this was how the rest of my life was going to be. But those who know me will tell you that I'm never one to stick with the status quo. Things were beginning to become predictable, and it was time for me to start figuring out what I wanted to do when my kids were in school. I spent a lot of time thinking about it, and kept coming back to my experiences with nurses during my deliveries and subsequent minor surgeries for each of my children. In each of those moments, it was a nurse who stood by my side. Nurses supported me when I needed it, educated me when I needed knowledge, and provided a constant presence and shoulder to lean on when I was worrying about my children. I wanted to be that person. I wanted to be that trusted. I wanted to be that valuable an influence on people's lives, knowing at the end of the day that I really had made a difference.

So I went off to nursing school, with what I now realize was absolutely zero idea of what I had gotten myself into. I think I really saw nursing as most of society sees it: hard, but not too hard; busy, but not too busy. I'd be able to sit at the side of my patient's bed all day and give them everything they needed. I'd be trusted by my patients and looked up to by the public. I'd make a pretty good wage for the work I did, and be able to get home at 3:30 pm every day to see my kids off of the school bus—right?! Once the classes and clinicals began, it was clear that there was much more to this world than I had known. Nursing school is hard—really hard! Clinicals and my work on the floor of a postpartum unit as a student tech are busy—really busy! Sit by the bedside of one patient all day? Nobody told me I'd have four to eight patients depending on the unit. I am trusted by my patients and the public, and they expect me to know the answers to every medical malady under the sun. My wages are nothing to shake a stick at, but my husband is continually amazed that nurses can hold someone's life in their hands and not come close to the salary of a computer software consultant. That said, the job has also been more satisfying than I ever thought possible. The schoolwork is quite challenging, but absolutely fascinating at the same time. I had wanted to make a difference in people's lives every day, and I really feel as though I've been able to do that.

One year of nursing school complete, and the old status quo feeling was starting to resurface. A friend talked me into running for treasurer of our university's Student Nurse Association (SNA). I was told that I would need to give an hour of my time a month, and I very seriously debated my ability to make that sort of commitment. Within two weeks,

NURSING VOICES

I was not only treasurer for my school SNA, but I was president of the state SNA. It was a crash course in what nursing is and what nursing can be—and the steps each of us can take to get it there. I learned about professional associations, legislative involvement, Robert's Rules of Order, resolutions, varying educational pathways, and so much more. I learned that I could have a personal influence on the image of nursing as a whole—positive or negative—both inside the profession and with the general public. I was hooked.

There is a part of nursing that I worry too many people never get to see. It is so easy to live your life, day to day, doing your job at the bedside and then going home. Our professors tell us that our job as a nurse is to be a patient advocate, but so many of us never realize that this advocacy role extends beyond the bedside care that we provide. We can and should play a role in legislative process. Who better to discuss patient care and medical and financial issues with legislators than a nurse who has sat at the bedside of a patient who cannot access needed care due to lack of adequate insurance? We can and should monitor the public's perception of nursing. It is wonderful that we are continually rated the most trusted profession in Gallup polling, but does the public realize how hard we work? Do we get paid properly? Are we provided with the tools that we need to safely lift patients without risk of self-injury? Do our patients think we're professionals, or do they see us as the background characters on a popular television show, or as sex objects with hypodermics? We can influence these perceptions. When we see a television show inaccurately portraying nurses, we can write them a letter or make a phone call and let them know our concern. We can become members of our professional organizations to show support for those lobbying on our collective behalf for laws to help improve our places of work as well as our patient outcomes. We can continue to read the latest research, working to implement evidence-based practice in our own places of work.

I am now a senior in my BSN nursing program, and I currently serve as president of the National Student Nurses Association. I also work, part-time, on the postpartum unit at one of my local hospitals. I have had the chance to be extremely involved in the professional image of nursing as compared to the typical nursing student, and to work alongside seasoned nurses at all levels of involvement. I have found that the best way to share these opportunities is to be involved myself, discuss them with everyone who will listen, and show others that their actions can move mountains as easily as anyone else's.

We hold the future image of nursing in our hands—and if that isn't a daunting responsibility, I'm not sure what is. We can choose to be grumpy and down about our careers when the patient load is high and resources are low, or we can work alongside management to open their eyes to issues on the floor and demonstrate ways to improve these conditions. As Mahatma Ghandi said, "We must be the change we wish to see in the world." This concept is a driving force for me, and one that I try regularly to communicate to my fellow students and coworkers. Life can be lived from the passenger seat, or you

NURSING VOICES

can choose to drive it and guide it yourself. Once you determine what changes you wish to see, you must live those changes.

The changes I would love to see in the future of nursing have certainly played a role in how I carry myself at school and at work. I want to see more nurses involved politically, so I share proposed bills and political involvement opportunities with students and coworkers. Explaining how they can play a role in the process is empowering, both for myself and for them! I want to see increases in evidence-based practice, so I read nursing journals and share the articles with those on my unit. I believe we have an incredible amount to learn from students and nurses around the globe, so I stay involved with international nursing organizations and take part in opportunities for cultural exchange whenever they are presented.

What our profession needs—or, really, desperately craves—is unity. Not every one of us is going to be a change leader, but if we can all actively support change through a professional organization, as a voting and professional body, we will be a force to be reckoned with. Improved nursing image brings improved pay, improved working conditions, and improved job satisfaction.

Do people at work and school think I'm nuts? Some of them definitely do. But over time, as they see the changes that can be made by being a part of the process, many have picked up a cause and jumped into the driver's seat. For those who choose not to participate in the process, the most common complaint is lack of time. As a mother of three, a full-time student, and one who struggled to decide whether I could spare an hour a month to be involved, I completely understand. That hour a month is comical now, but I wouldn't trade any of the experiences I have had. My response? You find time for what you are passionate about. We won't all be involved in the same issues, but if we can each find an issue that is personal to us in the nursing profession, and work to improve the problems and misperceptions, I have little doubt that nursing will continue to climb the ranks of highly respected professions—and we will continue to make immeasurable differences in our patients' lives.

Jenna Sanders is a senior BSN nursing student at the University of Saint Francis, in Fort Wayne, IN. She serves as president of the National Student Nurses' Association for the 2008–2009 term, having served in the past as NSNA vice president, Indiana Student Nurse Association president, and treasurer for her university's Student Nurse Association. Jenna plans to graduate in May 2009 with her BSN and a minor in business administration. Currently working as a student tech in the postpartum unit at a local hospital, her long-term goals include continued work in the labor and delivery and postpartum areas. Jenna has a passion for women's health and particularly enjoys patient education.

CHAPTER 3

Misperceptions of Image: How the Profession Is Perceived

By Karen L. Tomajan, MS, RN, BC, CNAA, CRRN

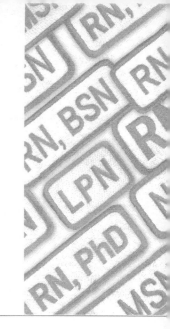

What Is a Public Image?

The image of nursing is important. Public image creates a framework by which others approach nursing as a profession, as well as each nurse individually. Image influences patient safety, resource allocation, public policy, recruitment into the profession, and other issues that have far-reaching consequences.

An image is a picture or concept in the minds of individuals or groups that influences their perceptions. The public image of nursing is the collective footprint of the profession created by the words and actions of the nearly three million nurses working today, plus the millions of nurses that have come before.

Nursing is a complex, dynamic, and diverse profession. The image of nursing is equally complex and dynamic. Nurses have been consistently ranked in Gallup public opinion polls as the most trusted professional group for eight of the past nine years, eclipsed only by firefighters in 2001. Despite this important acknowledgment of the honesty and trust of the public, the presence of nurses and nursing in the media speaking on healthcare issues is virtually absent. When nurses do speak out, it tends to be nurses in leadership or advanced practice positions, not bedside staff members discussing their important work (Buresh 2006; Woodhull Report 1998). When nursing issues are presented, the topics reflect problems: the nurse shortage, staffing ratios, or workplace issues. This problem focus does not promote a public understanding of what nurses do (Buresh 2006).

Why the Public Image of Nursing Is Important

This is an exciting time in healthcare. Never before has the role of the nurse been so pivotal to our patients, our employing agencies, or our profession. While the issues we face in healthcare are critical, we are an industry in flux. The opinions of nurses are important and valued. Presenting a balanced view of the nurse's role and contribution to healthcare is essential. The winds of change are evident, and it is important that nurses are primed and ready to assume the leadership roles necessary to advocate for a healthcare system focused on the needs of those we serve, to promote responsible resource allocation, to utilize the strengths and abilities of each occupational group to its full capacity, and to ensure patient safety and quality patient outcomes. The impact of nursing's image comes to bear in several important ways.

Resource allocation

Funding for healthcare, whether at the organizational or governmental level, is dependent on a common understanding of the needs of the population and the professional group making the request. Unless the contribution of the professional nurse is clearly articulated, funding for nursing could be jeopardized. From the nursing unit budget for staffing, training, equipment, and supplies, to the national budget for nursing research and scholarships, knowledge of what nurses do and what they contribute is vitally linked to the allocation of limited resources.

Influence on public policy

Healthcare issues are commonly addressed through legislation that moves the healthcare agenda into law. Unfortunately, multiple competing groups are involved, often advocating positions that are viewed as self-serving. Nursing opinion is viewed by legislators as balanced and objective because nurses focus on the impact of potential legislation on the public, with little opportunity for personal gain. For this reason, the opinion of the nurse is valued by legislators seeking to understand healthcare issues.

In addition to the legislative process, nurses influence public policy through professional associations, appointments to boards, commissions, task forces, and committees. Nurses also exert influence on public policy through presentations and written communication in the form of letters or white papers.

Recruitment into the profession

A growing concern is the evolving nursing workforce shortage, expected to peak in the next 10 years. This shortage will have monumental effects on healthcare, as it will hit at the same time as increased demands for healthcare by aging baby boomers, the largest segment of the U.S. population. Many initiatives are underway to address this crisis at the local, state, and national levels. Over the next few years, strategies to recruit individuals into nursing as well as retain practicing nurses will be vital to maintain the capacity of the healthcare system.

In order to recruit the best and brightest into nursing, it is also essential that students, teachers, and counselors have a more objective view of the role of the registered nurse. The traditional view, focused on the virtues of nurses as caring, compassionate workers, does not accurately portray the academic rigor required to become a nurse. The role of the nurse is fuzzy with regard to what we actually do. As nurses, we all know that nursing is based on hard science and tough academics, but the public does not. Nursing is not an academic major that just any student can complete successfully. However, students with the capacity for nursing are often directed to other, more "prestigious" careers, with nursing promoted as a "fallback" major—if at all. This "fuzzy" view of nursing has been created, in part, by an emphasis on the softer side of nursing. Taglines such as "the importance of a nurse's touch" or "a message of caring" reflect only one side of the nurse's role. A stronger focus on the expertise required to save lives through the application of hard science would go a long way to help recruit students with the requisite cognitive and interpersonal skills necessary to succeed in this career field. It is important to project a balanced professional image that reflects the level of education and autonomy that nurses actually possess.

Interdisciplinary relationships

Although nurses' autonomous role is incredibly important and should not be understated, the reality is that much of the nurse's work is accomplished in an interdisciplinary environment. In order to fulfill the requirements for coordination of care and advocacy for the needs of the patient, professional respect is essential.

Interdisciplinary relationships are built one person at a time on the collective foundation of relationships between occupational groups over the course of years. Patient care is best served by nurses with strong, assertive communication skills who are able to establish collegiality that is focused on patients and patient care.

Patient trust

We serve individuals with complex healthcare needs in vulnerable situations. In order to provide effective care, the nurse must establish a trusting relationship with patients, families, and significant others. The public image of nurses as trusted professionals provides an important backdrop for these relationships; however, the factors at play in the moment add other dimensions. Through consistency and skill, this relationship is crafted moment to moment, from nurse to nurse, and remains fluid and dynamic during the entire encounter. The patient's previous encounters are brought to the current situation as well, adding further complexity to the situation.

Morale within the profession

One of the most crucial requirements for retaining excellent, knowledgeable, experienced nurses in the profession, and most importantly at the bedside, is improving morale. Low morale has serious repercussions on the ability to recruit and retain the best and brightest.

Recently a student related that she had heard from practicing nurses in several clinical settings, "Get out while you still have time!" Surprisingly, this is not an isolated situation for this one nursing student in this particular community. Nursing students across the country are encountering similar attitudes.

It is important for nurses in every setting to work with administrators to improve the working environment by articulating their concerns and working collaboratively to address the issues. We have a responsibility as professionals to help bring new nurses into healthy work environments.

Increasing complexity of healthcare

Another key aspect of nurse morale is the increasing complexity of care in most settings. Changes in healthcare funding in concert with changing patient populations have resulted in greater demands on the nurse and increased workloads. Patient needs are more complex, and yet lengths of stay are shorter. This cascade of events has resulted in an increased intensity of the work of nurses. Nurses experience greater job stress than in the past, and at times exhibit collective behaviors that have contributed to a stilted image of nurses as unhappy, vindictive individuals who complain or attack one another. Reactions to this increased level of stress vary from agency to agency. In some settings empowered nurses have worked with administration to develop acceptable strategies to improve the work environment. In other settings, nurses have turned to third-party agents—namely, unions—in the hopes of addressing their concerns. In still other agencies the issues go unaddressed, resulting in demoralized nurses with little hope of seeing improvements.

Nursing's role as sentinel

In the last several years, the issue of "failure to rescue" has been raised in both the popular press and professional healthcare literature (Aleccia 2008, Davies 2004, Clarke 2003). Failure to rescue is defined by Clarke (2003) as "the clinical inability to save a hospitalized patient's life when he experiences a complication not present on admission." Clark describes the critical role of the nurse as such: "[The] first to detect early signs of possible complications, their vigilance makes timely rescue responses more likely . . . rescuing the patient means they must be able to mobilize hospital resources quickly, including the ability to bring physicians to the bedside. Nurses' status within a hospital—as reflected by their credibility and rapport with physicians and the support received from hospital administration—influences the extent to which they can do so." The nurse's sentinel role is vital to patient safety, yet is not well understood by the public, administrators, legislators, and other policy makers (Clarke 2003). Maintaining a positive nursing image is vital to patient safety.

It is important that nurses take every opportunity to articulate their contribution to positive healthcare outcomes in every possible venue. Everyday questions such as "What do you do for a living?" and "What did you do today?" provide nurses with an opportunity to tell the story of what we do and to educate others on the vital role of the professional nurse. We recognize changes in patient status, prevent complications, promote positive patient outcomes, and act to save lives. Our roles are active, not passive; proactive, not reactive. The protective role of the nurse has been described as that of the "sentinel" of healthcare.

In 2002, The Joint Commission, the regulatory agency that accredits most hospitals, published a study on the shortage of nurses, which stated that "nearly every person's healthcare experience involves the contribution of a registered nurse" (The Joint Commission 2002). Birth and death and all the various forms of care in between are attended by the knowledge, support, and comforting of nurses. Few professions offer such a special opportunity for meaningful work. Yet this country is facing a growing shortage of registered nurses. When there are too few nurses, patient safety is threatened and healthcare quality is diminished.

How Negative Stereotypes Affect Nursing's Image

When looking at the media representations of nurses, it is clear that the nurse rarely is portrayed accurately. From television dramas and comedies to movies and beyond, there is concern within the profession that negative stereotypes of nurses undermine our credibility and create confusion about the real role and contribution of the professional nurse (Center for Nursing Advocacy 2008). Chapter 10 discusses the media stereotypes in greater detail, but a brief overview of the various misperceptions of nursing includes the following:

Angel of mercy – Nurses are sometimes represented as selfless, caring individuals who subjugate their own needs to those they serve. This image may be helped along by the belief that nurses have a "calling" to the profession. This image tells only a part of the story, undermining the important sentinel role of the nurse, who is educated in science and working to save lives, prevent complications, and promote positive patient outcomes.

Naughty nurse – An image of the nurse in a short miniskirt with her blouse unbuttoned and cleavage exposed is another beloved media stereotype. The "naughty nurse" is often portrayed as "ditzy" as well, undermining the requirements for nurses to be educated in the sciences and to think critically. This image undermines the credibility of nursing as a serious profession, as well as the credibility of each individual nurse.

Nurse Ratched – A prominent character from the Academy Award–winning movie *One Flew Over the Cuckoo's Nest*, Nurse Ratched was a sadistic psychiatric nurse who abused her professional power to break the will of a group of patients on a psychiatric unit. Since this movie's release in 1975, uttering the name of Nurse Ratched conjures up a controlling, manipulative individual. Professional nursing is built on the ability to establish a trusting relationship with our patients. Any negative stereotype that undermines the ability to establish trust undermines our profession.

Handmaiden – The handmaiden stereotype embraces only the dependent role of the registered nurse. This image of the traditional nurse involves an overemphasis on following doctors' orders. The reality is that professional nurses cannot possibly care for their patients effectively without exercising the independent functions of their role. This inaccurate portrayal of both the nurse and the physician undermines the credibility of both professional groups, and creates confusion for the public.

A recent study of the public perception of nursing careers (Donelan et al. 2008) reinforced previous findings that nurses are held in high public regard. This study asked people to say the first words that came to mind when hearing the term registered nurse: 32% responded with terms such as knowledgeable, educated professionals and 43% responded with terms such as caring, compassionate, dedicated, and trustworthy. Thirteen percent identified nurses as helpers or assistants to doctors, indicating the handmaiden perception. While 16% spoke about nurses being overworked, underpaid, and stressed, which ties into the perception of nursing as an attractive career.

In addition, the affect of media exposure on the public's respect for nurses was studied, and the majority of respondents asserted that television and movie portrayals of nurses were more likely to have no effect on them than to have a positive or negative effect. This study lends credence to the important role nurses play in forming public opinions of our profession. It recognizes the potential we have in changing public perceptions. It also goes some way to dispel some of the concerns we have had about the portrayal of nurses in the media. While more exposure to what nurses actually do would have huge benefit, the misrepresentation has not been as detrimental as may have been feared.

Are other professions concerned about public image?

Surprisingly, most professional groups are concerned about how they are perceived by the public. A Google search on "public image" reveals numerous occupational groups struggling to improve their public images. For instance, the North American Actuarial Organization set out to promote a public image campaign to raise awareness of the services their members provide, and to promote a more dynamic public image. Chemists struggle with the stereotypic image of the "mad scientist" and the shadow of Dr. Frankenstein. The American Society of Civil Engineers have a model to promote civil engineering based on a four-step plan to increase awareness; increase appreciation; improve understanding; and promote action, which includes media relations, promoting recruitment into the profession, and advancing public affairs through grants and training. Overall, not a bad plan!

As important as it is to work toward improving or updating the public image of nursing, it is perhaps more important to work toward improving the self-image of the nurse. The day-to-day behaviors exhibited by nurses in their work and how their work is represented in their descriptions of what they do are what reinforce or contradict the images projected by the media. Because of the vast diversity among nurses, public image has the potential to be flexible and to truly reflect our diversity.

Efforts to Promote a More Accurate Public Image

Over the past 20 years, several important national initiatives have been undertaken to promote a more accurate public image of nursing. (One of them, the Center for Nursing Advocacy, will be discussed in depth in Chapter 10.) The focus of these efforts has been to increase the awareness of the importance of image, and to educate nurses on using the media to promote nursing and initiate a more active media presence. These initiatives resulted in some success, but more importantly they have helped nurses to more fully understand the impact the culture of their profession has had on public image, and flushed out a reluctance to actively engage in opportunities to tout personal accomplishments. Even when actively assisted to engage media interaction, nurses still are uncomfortable with the active promotion of the contributions of nursing and nurses to the healthcare system, particularly when emphasizing the independent functions of the professional nurse. This reluctance to take the microphone, camera, or stage to promote the contributions of our profession has had the deleterious effect of an inaccurate public image of the professional nurse's role, as well as an underreporting of the positive impact nursing has on the healthcare system.

Nurses of America project

The Nurses of America project, funded by the Pew Charitable Trust, began in 1989. Suzanne Gordon and Bernice Buresh, both respected journalists, were engaged to educate nurses and nursing leaders in media relations. Though active for only a few years, this project has had a lasting impact on the nursing profession. Many nurses were trained in media relations, but more importantly, through the longstanding relationship the consulting journalists have maintained with members of the profession, the project's influence remains to this day. The book *From Silence to Voice: What Nurses Know and Must Communicate to the Public* is based on Gordon and Buresh's work with this project, and remains an outstanding resource on the public image of nursing.

Woodhull Study on nursing and the media

In 1997, the Sigma Theta Tau International Honor Society of Nursing commissioned the Woodhull Study on the representation of nursing in the media. The study found that nurses and nursing were referenced in less than 3% of hundreds of stories on healthcare. The final recommendations included increasing nursing presence through more active media relations. The final report, published in 1999, was entitled "Healthcare's Invisible Partner."

American Nurses Association

In response to the Woodhull study, in 1999 the American Nurses Association (ANA) produced a toolkit and videotape to train nurse leaders in media relations. The toolkit was used to provide media training for ANA leaders at the state and national levels.

A number of state nurses associations are working to advance the image of nursing within their respective states. For example, the New York State Nurses Association spent 2007 focusing on nursing image. The Mid-Ohio District Nurses Association, an affiliate of the Ohio Nurses Association, developed pocket cards as a reference for nurses. These cards define the role of the registered nurse and can be distributed to managers,

legislators, or anyone else. For more information about the card, contact the association through its Web site *www.modna.org*.

ANCC Magnet Recognition Program®

The American Nurses Credentialing Center (ANCC) Magnet Recognition Program® (MRP) has made a tremendous contribution to the image of nursing. Organizations applying for MRP designation are required to address how the contributions of nurses are recognized, describe the relationship between nursing and other departments and disciplines, demonstrate the impact of nurses in nontraditional roles on the organization and nursing image, and describe the image of nursing in the community. Advertising materials must be submitted and reviewed to ensure nursing is promoted respectfully and accurately. During the site visit, staff members validate all submitted materials (ANCC 2008).

Campaign for Nursing's Future

Sponsored by Johnson & Johnson, the Campaign for Nursing's Future began in 2002 to promote nursing as a career option. This campaign provides complimentary recruitment brochures, posters, and videos. The intent of this campaign was applauded by the nursing community. Coming at a time when the full impact of the nursing shortage was just becoming clear, Johnson & Johnson provided a real service to healthcare by providing the resources necessary to launch a national campaign at the local level. The initial tagline, "the importance of a nurse's touch," was a classic example of representing only the softer side of nursing, and consequently the message of the campaign received mixed reviews from nursing advocacy groups.

National Student Nurses' Association

If there are any questions regarding the commitment of the next generation of nurses to upholding and promoting the public image of nursing, fear not! The National Student Nurses' Association has had an Image of Nursing program since 1993. The goal of this program is to dispel misconceptions the public may have of nurses and the profession by educating nursing students on professionalism and promoting a positive public image. Each year, state and school chapters are encouraged to develop projects to address nursing image issues and then apply to the national organization for recognition.

Professional associations

Much of the work done to advance nursing image at the national level has been sponsored by nursing professional organizations, such as the American Nurses Association, Sigma Theta Tau, and the National Student Nurses Association. In Chapter 2, Cohen reviewed the results of her survey of nurse's perceptions of the image of nursing and examined results to the question "What do you think the individual nurse can do to help shape a more realistic image of nursing?" Only 23% of respondents identified membership in professional organizations as a solution. Consider this in relation to the fact that only about 20% of all nurses belong to a professional organization, despite the fact that more than 50 nursing organizations exist. One question to consider is whether only those nurses who belong to an association recognized the contribution our associations have made to advance the public image of nursing, particularly at the national level.

Membership in professional associations has a positive effect on the profession, as well as on individual nurses. If more nurse belonged to professional associations, these groups would have greater resources to continue their efforts on behalf of the profession.

REFERENCES

Alecia, J. (2008). "Before Code Blue: Who's minding the patient?" Available at *www.msnbc.msn.com/id/24002334/*.

American Nurses Association. (1999). ANA Media Relations and You. Washington, D.C.: American Nurses Publishing.

American Nurses Credentialing Center. (2008). "Program overview." *Available at www.nursecredentialing.org/Magnet.*

Buresh, B., and Gordon, S. (2006). *From Silence to Voice, What Nurses Know and Must Communicate to the Public* (2nd Ed.). New York: Cornell University Press.

Clarke, S.P., Aiken, L.A. (2003). "Failure to rescue: Needless deaths are prime examples of the need for more nurses at the bedside." *American Journal of Nursing* 103(1): 42-47.

Davies, D. (2004). "Fatal medical errors said to be more widespread." *Wall Street Journal.* July 24, 2004.

Donelan, K., Buerhaus, P., DesRoches, C., Dittus, R., and Dutwin, D. (2008). "Public perceptions of nursing careers: The influence of the media and nursing shortages." *Nursing Economic$* 26(3): 142-165.

Gallup (2008). "Honesty/Ethics in professions." Available at *www.gallup.com/poll/1654/Honesty-Ethics-Professions.aspx*.

Gordon, S. (2005). *Nursing Against the Odds: How Health Care Cost Cutting, Media Stereotypes and Medical Hubris Undermine Nurses and Patient Care*. New York: Cornell University Press.

McClure, M, and Hinshaw, A.S. (2002). *Magnet Hospitals Revisited: Attraction and Retention of Professional Nurses*. Washington, D.C.: American Nurses Publishing.

Sigma Theta Tau. (1998). "Health Care's Invisible Partner: Woodhull Study on Nursing and the Media." Available at *www.nursingsociety.org*.

Sullivan, E.J. (2003). *Becoming Influential: A Guide for Nurses*. Upper Saddle River, NJ: Prentice Hall.

National Student Nurses Association (2007). "Image of nursing projects planning guide." Available at *www.nsna.org*.

The Center for Nursing Advocacy. (2008). "Frequently asked questions about nurses and nursing." Available at *www.nursingadvocacy.org*.

The Joint Commission. (2002). "Health care at the crossroads: Strategies for addressing the evolving nursing crisis." Available at *www.jointcommission.org*.

Tomajan, K. (2007). "Facilitating staff development." Online nurse manager evidence-based nursing course for Sigma Theta Tau International. Available at *www.nursingknowledge.org*.

CHAPTER 4

Autonomy, Power, and Image: Steps to Take Toward Empowerment

By Kathleen Bartholomew, RN, MN

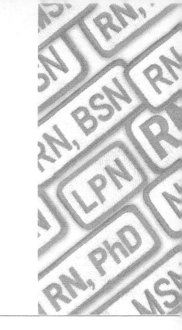

After reading this chapter, the participant will be able to:

✔ Discuss the connection between power and image

✔ Explain how nursing autonomy contributes to professionalism

"Be a fountain, not a drain." – Rex Hudler

Autonomy

Autonomy and power are two forces that greatly affect our nursing image. Up until now, we've been discussing external factors such as wardrobe, language, and behaviors. This chapter focuses on the internal forces that contribute to creating image. Think of a projector. Autonomy brings the picture we are projecting into focus, and power produces enough light to project that image on the screen. Without a clear sense of self, the image we portray is fuzzy. Without power, the image we portray is dim.

Trying to be powerful without autonomy would be like trying to hold water without a vessel. Autonomy is the amount of control that we have over our practice. Autonomy is our holding power, and it requires a strong sense of self. It is also a well-known fact that the more autonomy you have, the higher your job satisfaction. How much control do nurses actually have over their practice?

For example, a charge nurse decides that she needs five nurses to adequately staff the next shift—but the staffing office says she can only have four. A surgical nurse foresees the possibility of complications in a third-day postop patient and recommends to the physician that the patient stay another day—but the physician discharges the patient home anyway. The nurse notices on the fourth postop day that the patient has not had a bowel movement—but she can't give Maalox or even a suppository without calling the doctor.

Many of our day-to-day experiences place the nurse in a dependent, rather than an autonomous, position. Furthermore, the degree of autonomy we experience often changes depending on whose patient we are caring for, or the time of day—or both. This variability produces uncertainty and can be traced back to the roots of our profession, when the nurse's role was constructed to work under the supervision of a physician.

In his book *Beyond Caring* (1996), Daniel Chambliss identifies the three major directives inherent in nursing. He calls these "missions." A nurse must be a caring individual, a professional, and a subordinate member of the organization. Unfortunately, "The directives conflict: be caring and yet be a professional, be subordinate and yet responsible, be diffusely accountable for a patient's well being, and yet oriented to the hospital as an economic employer."

> My patient had his right hand amputated—but the chart was marked *"short stay"* so I was expected to discharge him within 23 hours. Is this the best decision for the patient or the institution? It will take another day at least until I can even begin to implement my nursing diagnosis of *"alteration in body image."* The conflict leaves me in a difficult position.

Every day nurses live out these conflicts. Every day brings competing priorities: get your work done,

do it right, and also take the time to be caring and attentive. But caring is devalued in today's health/business system, where efficiency and productivity are the dominant values. The engagement of one heart to the next cannot be measured or charted—it is an intangible. Today, the amount of time the average hospital nurse has to develop and nourish a relationship with a patient is gravely compromised and still dwindling. Caring is an intrinsic value of nursing and we all know it. Society expects it, and patients take it for granted that their nurse, a perfect stranger, will care for them with the attentiveness of a close relative.

A professional is frequently viewed as clinically detached—this is exactly how doctors are trained. If a physician walks into a room where I am engaged in comforting the patient, my actions are viewed as "soft, complimentary, and a nice feminine attribute." If a physician comes in to the patient's room and I coolly relay a list of critical assessments, I am viewed as a professional who is "really on top of the situation." The doctor represents the perceptions of society. Unfortunately, society cannot understand the role and challenges inherent in being both *caring and a professional*.

Caring is precisely the engagement necessary for not only thorough diagnostics, but for creating the optimal healing environment and facilitating recovery. With highly trained powers of observation and a vast knowledge base obtained by years of experience, nurses skillfully assess and implement a plan of care that is revised multiple times each hour *while* genuinely caring for their patients. This is exactly the message that every nurse must communicate to his or her patients, families, and the public. "If nurses continue to remain silent, the competitive market will find someone else who can fill in workplace gaps related to the nursing shortage"

(Needleman et al 2000). In fact, this is already happening, as Ohio has passed a law making the educational requirement for passing medications in a nursing home either a GED or high school diploma.

An unarticulated conflict is much more damaging to our esteem than an obvious one. The reason for discussing these conflicts is to raise awareness of their presence and effect. Most nurses take the above conflicts as 'part of the job,' and fail to see how these daily conundrums chip away at our sense of autonomy and self-esteem. An undertow is more powerful than a wave. So much conflict surrounds our most basic "mission" that it makes it difficult to establish a positive sense of identity or a clearly defined role. These subtle cultural forces work to keep our self-esteem low, reinforcing nurses' feelings of powerlessness. Raising awareness of these internal role conflicts, however, allows us to intervene and change course. Now that we have identified where the undertow pulls us down, we can chart a different course.

Five steps toward a positive identify

Susan Jo Roberts proposes five stages to attaining a positive identity: unexamined acceptance, awareness, connection, synthesis, and political action. These stages provide a framework for attaining a positive self-image or identity. In the first stage, unexamined acceptance, we "accept the role of the nurse as subservient in the system." But in the second stage, awareness, we begin to understand the power grid and the myths. In this stage we tend to take sides and believe nurses are always right and others are wrong. Because of the increased pace of work, which results in less time to reflect and bond with each other, many nurses are often caught in this particular stage. Characterized by complaining, this is the stage in which nurses frequently talk about how they have been wronged. When you hear these comments every day over a long period of time, you begin to think that's who you are. As I travel around the country speaking to nurses, I am convinced from their comments, that the majority are stuck in this phase.

In the third stage, connection, "nurses make a linkage to other nurses built on the beginning of a new self and professional identity." Nurses find other nurses who also share their vision of an emerging professional positive identity. Often they will join professional organizations to share new ideas and offer support to each other.

It is in the next stage, synthesis, that we feel our authentic self. "Anger turns into strategic efforts toward change" and nurses learn to appreciate each other's differences. Our new positive view of nursing is internalized, and we join interdisciplinary efforts with a renewed sense of energy, knowing what nursing has to offer.

The final stage is urgently needed: political action. In this stage, nurses are actively involved in the process of reform because of their genuine commitment to social change. The focus is on the broader issues of humanity, and nurses see and grasp the opportunity to "change the system that once oppressed them" (Roberts 2000).

TIP

Look at Figure 4.1, which describes professional identity development. Which stage best describes where you are today? Recognize that you can go back and forth between the stages and that they don't have to be followed in a rigid order.

FIGURE 4.1   IDENTITY DEVELOPMENT FOR NURSING

Unexamined Acceptance	Awareness	Connection	Synthesis	Political Action
Acceptance of roles of nurses	Awakening to a sense of injustice	Affiliation with nursing groups	Internalizes new positive view of nursing	Committment to change
Unquestioned belief in the power structure	Nurses are always right, others are wrong	Dependent on support of other nurses for new ideas	Evaluates others on an individual basis	Actively involved
Belief that physicians should control the system	Overwhelmed by sense of having been wronged	Viewed as strident and rigid.	Increase in interdisciplinary involvement	Broad scope of activities to further social justice
Internalized negative view of nursing	Seeks out other nurses for support	Affirmation of positive identity as a nurse	Strategic approach to problem solving	
			Nurses are different but equal	

Source: Susan Jo Roberts, DNSc, ANP. (2000). "Development of a positive professional identity: Liberating oneself from the oppressor within." Advances in Nursing Science 22 (4): 71-82. Reprinted with permission.

Power

Nurses in Cohen's image survey asked, "How did we lose our professionalism?" Certainly, there have been pockets of professionalism in nursing throughout the years, but did we ever really have it?

Yes, at least a few nurses did. But professionalism was never fully disseminated throughout nursing. It takes a long time to create a culture of collegiality and professionalism, but that is what this book is all about: getting everyone on board, connecting the dots, and connecting the "pockets of professionalism" until we clearly define and see a new image. We are working toward an image of the compassionate, highly skilled nurse professional who is held in great esteem, protected and supported by the greater society that can clearly articulate the nurse's role. To do this, we begin by addressing recent concerns of nurses about professionalism.

There is a perception among many nurses that in the last decade we have become less professional. When asked about what constitutes this

 The Image of Nursing

lack of professionalism, nurses respond with specific examples:

- "It's a free-for-all with our dress code—and embarrassing to witness some of my coworkers' attire."

- "It just seems like there's a lot more backstabbing and gossip on the floor than there used to be."

- "Our state doesn't require continuing education anymore, so no one bothers."

- "The work ethic around here has changed—it's all about getting the tasks finished now."

We see and hear these comments amongst us, yet struggle to understand the bigger picture. What is happening here? What larger story do these comments portray? There are many excellent books on the history of nursing and the factors that have contributed to our image of handmaiden rather than professional. In this section, we will focus on factors that have contributed to the perception and feeling of loss surrounding professionalism, specifically during the last decade: an emphasis on the science of nursing, a lack of solidarity, cost cutting due to managed care, human adaptability, and the nursing shortage.

Science of nursing

As a relatively new profession, nursing has been focused on proving to the world that it is a valid profession. Less than 20 years ago, nursing was still being referred to as a "semi-profession." Therefore, we poured our energy and attention into research and the science of nursing practice to demonstrate to the world that nursing is a true profession. Today, this knowledge base provides a foundation for a respectable practice.

Lack of solidarity

We lack solidarity, and any group that lacks solidarity can't mobilize its resources. We operated (and continue to operate) as an oppressed group. Oppressed groups are those that live and work with another group that has more power (e.g., physicians, administration). Oppressed groups lack self-esteem, autonomy, accountability, and power. When there "isn't enough to go around," the group starts competing within itself for the scarce resources available. The most obvious example of this is the fact that after 100 years we still can't agree on the basic educational requirements necessary for RN licensure. A more general example is when nurses do not get along or form cliques on their units—both examples of horizontal hostility.

Cost cutting

Cost cutting in the late 1990s decreased the financial resources available to nursing across the board. Educator positions were slashed, and managers were given multiple units to manage *and* fewer resources. Multihospital networks were formed to generate greater bargaining power as a response to managed care, which was designed to change physician and hospital behavior. "Merger mania" ensued and swept the industry in the 1990s, and this vast restructuring resulted in fewer resources to nurses (Weinberg). All this created an additional workload for almost every nurse in an institution, created more stress, and reinforced nurses' feelings of powerlessness.

Human adaptability

When changes are slow and incremental, they are not noticed by human beings. The metaphor of the frog is used to explain this theory: When you throw a frog in hot water, he jumps out right away. When you throw a frog in cold water and turn the temperature up slowly, he stays where he is, even as he boils to death. More technology means more pharmaceuticals, more patients with multiple admitting diagnoses and chronic diseases, learning more new skill sets (such as computerized charting), and a decreased length of stay. Floating to an oncology unit this summer, I was shocked to open the medication record and find 35 scheduled medications were due to a patient on my shift—and I only recognized 18! How hot is the water for nurses? Recent research documents that the number of tasks required has increased, the time to complete them has decreased, and work complexity has increased due to these factors (Nelson, Gordon).

In addition, nursing leaders have been very busy conveying the seriousness of the global nursing shortage to the public and the government. They have been spending a great deal of time and energy advocating for more nursing resources for students while struggling with a dwindling faculty work force. Add to this increased regulatory pressures and it is easy to see how difficult it would be for any profession to address these challenges while putting energy toward raising their level of professionalism!

What we can control, however, is how we respond to these pressures. As I used to tell my staff, "There are things we can control and things we can't. Let's focus on what we can." Raising the bar for professionalism begins by understanding how we use our personal power—and how we lose it.

Personal Power

Personal power starts with awareness. What drains you? What are the situations that day after day seem to suck all your energy and strength? Being able to identify where your personal power takes your energy is the first step to empowerment, because then you can plug the hole.

> "Gretchen is always complaining—and she's always so negative. I'm tired of hearing it, so I just ignore it."
>
> "I'm sick of doing all the work while the nursing assistants sit at the hubs doing nothing."
>
> "The staffing ratio here is unacceptable—but there's no use going to the manager begging for resources. Nothing ever changes."

Power is the ability to act or produce an effect. Every time we tolerate an unacceptable situation, we drain our personal power reservoir a little more. Learning how to tackle these situations professionally is a new skill for many of us because the most common way to learn is by imitation, and many of the professional styles we have witnessed have been far from optimal.

The reverse is also true. Every time we handle a previously disempowering situation, we gain personal power, and consequently our sense of self-esteem increases. One by one, as the competency skills and self-esteem of nurses increase, our group sense of self-esteem also will rise.

TIP

Try this exercise: List the top two situations that drain you of energy/power. Stop tolerating the situations and instead think of ways to permanently resolve them.

What Does Power Have to Do With Image?

Everything! If the staffing levels are inappropriate and unsafe on your unit and you *feel* like you have no power, you won't be moved to take action. If you tolerate an unacceptable situation, then you end up feeling powerless.

Everyone has personal power, but some of us use it better than others. Acting in a different way is always a risk, and taking risks takes courage. Our jobs are our livelihoods, and after working for an organization for years, many would rather tolerate the status quo than put their jobs at risk.

What keeps us from acting? What keeps us from our "power"?

Fear. Silence. Fear of speaking up, or fear of being rejected, or of retaliation, or alienation. One common characteristic of powerless (i.e., oppressed) groups is that they will tolerate a situation rather than rocking the boat, because speaking out can make the group more vulnerable by increasing its visibility, thereby putting the entire group in danger. This knowledge is rarely verbalized, but instead remains deeply embedded within the culture of nursing. Rather than feeling more empowered as tenure in nursing increases, one study showed that nurses with 1–5 years of experience felt more empowered than nurses who had 6–15 years of experience (Kuokkanen et. al 2002). One explanation is that the more we are "socialized" into the nursing profession,

and the more experiences of "what's the use?" we have, the more our powerlessness is reinforced.

What systems or processes keep the nurse in a position of powerlessness?

Mandatory overtime, feelings of powerlessness and victimization from horizontal hostility or ineffective/authoritarian leadership, and an inability to deal with conflict or resolve difficult issues are a few of the major forces that work to keep your power suppressed. By raising our awareness level about these particular situations and developing an action plan, we can (and will) increase our personal power.

Authoritarian or ineffective leadership: When staff members ask for help and support and do not even receive an acknowledgment of their problem from management, they feel hopeless to change the situation. A failure to acknowledge the needs and concerns of staff causes feelings of disempowerment.

If you have tried to resolve an issue on the floor and were unsuccessful, the next step should be to go to your manager for help. Unfortunately, I sometimes hear comments like, "You don't understand; she's one of them," or "There's no use, I've already tried." These are common phrases used by anyone who feels that they are powerless.

Use the chain of command. Go to the director and, without using names or blaming, clearly state the issue, your efforts to resolve the issue, and the outcome thus far. Ask for the support you need.

Inability to deal with conflict/resolve difficult issues: This results in a profound feeling of powerlessness as well. In fact, one researcher found a direct correlation between burnout and conflict: learning how to handle difficult situations will decrease our feelings of burnout (Farrell 2001). Therefore, an entire chapter in this book (Chapter 6) will be devoted to specific strategies and tools for handling difficult situations.

Personal and Professional Power

In Chapter 1, Shelley Cohen asks, "Who took over the decision [about our image] while nursing was arguing amongst itself?" The answer to this question sheds a lot of light on nursing's image challenges.

Nursing has been "arguing amongst itself" because

> After a conference, a participant asked to speak to me in private. For 10 minutes she explained her disastrous work situation. When finally I could speak, I said, *"Why do you stay? Why don't you apply for a job at another hospital?"* The look on her face was both surprise and resistance. *"Why, I could never do that,"* she responded slowly.
>
> *"Why?"* I asked. *"Why can't you?"* This nurse had experienced so many negative situations where she felt helpless to solve the problem that she actually believed that she was helpless, that there was no way out. This is perceived helplessness. Without another word, she sat down, still struggling to come up with an answer to my question.

infighting is a known characteristic of groups of people who have no power. As long ago as 1983, Sandra Roberts pointed out the similarities between nursing and other oppressed groups. She noted that when people cannot direct their power upward, they overpower each other. Unfortunately, the healthcare model in the United States is a business model, which by its very nature implies that the primary focus and dominant power is money. The budget dictates everything. Nursing is constantly overruled by administration, insurance companies' dictates, physicians, and even our own "health" care system. How do we know that nurses are oppressed in this system?

- A PhD in nursing will get you a job offer of $47,000 per year—half of what a master's in business would make.

- The charge nurse, who is the *only* person qualified to staff a shift, has no authority or say in how many nurses are needed.

- When the CEO calls the annual budget meeting, he or she doesn't ask the CNO for his or her needs first and then balance the institution's finances around bedside needs.

- There are temporary CNO companies. What other profession has a temp agency for its highest office?

- Nurses are responsible for the outcomes, but not the resources.

Roberts did more than point out the problem; she showed us the solutions as well. In order to unite as a profession, we need to "lift the veil" and raise our individual and collective self-esteem. "Lifting the veil" means raising your awareness to the point where you can know and understand that the forces that suppress you are a perceived helplessness—a learned helplessness—acquired by our acculturation process into the society of nursing. The show is over and the game is up when we see that in everyday situations there is both an opportunity and a responsibility to act—in other words, to produce an effect, which is the definition of power!

I floated to the Short Stay unit last week, where a patient was abusing the nurses and blatantly refusing the plan of care. The physician was made aware of these behaviors and "said something" to the patient during rounds. Not more than 30 minutes after the physician left the floor, the patient began acting out again. The nurse was frustrated as she complained to her coworker about what a horrible day it was going to be—again. I suggested that she obtain a Behavioral Contract, which would clearly outline the acceptable and nonacceptable behaviors and result in discharge if not followed.

Her response: *"He [the physician] will never go for that."* I encouraged the nurse and asked her to take care of herself and challenge her assumption that she could do nothing about this situation. With coaching, she called the physician and asked him to come back to the floor to fill out the contract with the patient.

Actual Power vs. Perceived Power

Our perception is our reality: Change your perception, and you change your world.

One example of "perceived" power is the relationship between a nurse and physician. The nurse may disagree with a physician, but doesn't put the energy out to confront him or her, because the perception is that the physician has more power—or that the nurse doesn't have enough power over the situation. This is demonstrated through comments such as "That's just the way he is," "She's never going to change," and so on.

In the previous example, I called this nurse to draw on her actual power, instead of her misperceived total lack of power. How do you think that nurse felt after the phone call? What do you think she will do the next time this situation occurs?

TIP

Identify a situation that happened in your workplace that could have turned out differently if you had a coach. Be that coach the next time!

Unions are another example of "perceived" power. Doctors and lawyers don't belong to unions, but powerless groups such as teachers, nurses, and service workers are represented by unions. This is because all of these groups are oppressed, meaning that their experiences taught them that they could not rally themselves against the status quo. Unions came into existence for a reason: Rights were being abused and people felt powerless. When we belong to a union we feel more powerful, and we feel a sense of protection and safety in representation. But this power is "perceived" power as opposed to "actual" power.

The goal of a union is *not* to increase the self-esteem and confidence of every nurse. If it were, then they would be out of business, because we wouldn't be oppressed anymore! This "perception" of power is what keeps the unions in business. To some degree, unions have helped improve our working conditions, but their primary goal is power and *not* empowerment.

If our sense of self and group esteem were to rise, we would realize that as a group we can accomplish anything. But we can't do this as a group until we can do it as individuals. We can be a strong and powerful force of almost three million voices strong—*if* we unite.

TIP

Join a professional nonunionized organization such as the American Nurses Association, Center for Nursing Advocacy, or the Center for American Nurses.

"There is nothing from outside that can endanger us. It will come from within."
—Beverly Malone, past ANA president

Actual power transforms. It changes your life in a moment; you know it and feel its effects immediately. When you confront a peer about something negative you overheard about yourself, you are exercising your power, and consequently your self-esteem meter rises. When you have a heart-to-heart talk with a doctor who has been a problem, and resolve the issue together, you feel a sense of strength and power. *This personal power is the hope of the nursing profession.*

From personal power comes professional power. When you advocate for safer staffing, use the chain of command instead of tolerating an unacceptable situation, help pass a bill that protects a vulnerable population, or advocate for higher education standards, you are representing the core values of our profession. If we take these steps, the public will eventually see who we are and what we do.

Professional power will increase our political power as we join together to make our voices heard: first a solo, then a duet, and then a choir, until everyone knows nursing's song. What are the lyrics? They are a Nightingale sonnet about our belief in ourselves, our profession, and humanity; about our desire to heal society by improving the health of all its members; about a group of people who in every interaction demonstrate that they value and honor *who they are and what they do!*

RECIPE FOR UNPROFESSIONALISM

Take a group of intelligent women without power whose value system is primarily service (compassionate, highly skilled, safe, quality care) and have them work in the opposite value system, where money is revered above everything. Then, put them in a position where they are responsible for the outcome, but not the resources; responsible to the patient, but also the institution; have autonomy, but only sometimes; where they are skilled and knowledgeable, but the person they work under every day never bothers to ask their opinion, acknowledge their work, or, often, even ask their name.

Eventually, this ambiguity will produce a great deal of uncertainty and stress. Keep telling them that the impossible amount of complex tasks required of them in a short amount of time is reasonable and doable so that they will berate themselves when they fall short—and each other as well (without even realizing that they are doing this.) Combine the disparity in values, uncertainty, stress, feelings of failure, and low self-esteem. Let this simmer shift after shift, week after week, and year after year until they burn out or leave, and the average age of the nurse climbs to 48, 49, 50 . . .

REFERENCES

Chambliss, D.F. (1996). *Beyond Caring: Hospitals, Nurses, and the Social Organization of Ethics*. Chicago: University Of Chicago Press.

Roberts, S.J. (2000). "Development of a positive professional identity: Liberating oneself from the oppressor within." Advances in Nursing Science 22 (4): 71–82.

Farrell, G. (2001)."From tall poppies to squashed weeds: Why don't nurses pull together more?" Journal of Advanced Nursing 35(1): 26–33.

Gordon, S. (2005). *Nursing Against the Odds: How Health Care Cost Cutting, Media Stereotypes and Medical Hubris Undermine Nurses and Patient Care.* New York: Cornell University Press.

Kuokkanen, L., Leino-Kilpi, H., Katajisto, J. (2002). "Do nurses feel empowered? Nurses' assessments of their own qualities and performance with regard to nurse empowerment." *Journal of Professional Nursing* 18(6): 328–35.

Needleman, J., Buerhaus, P., Mattke, S., Stewart, M. & Zelevinsky, K. (2002). "Nurse staffing and quality of care in hospitals in the United States." *The New England Journal of Medicine* 346 (22): 1715–1722.

Nelson, S. & Gordon, S. (2006) *The Complexities of Care: Nursing Reconsidered.* New York: Cornell University Press.

Weinberg, D. (2003). Code Green: *Money Driven Hospitals and the Dismantling of Nursing.* Ithaca, NY: Cornell University Press.

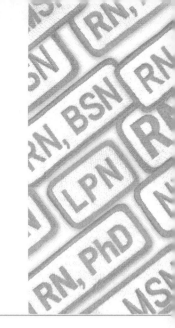

CHAPTER 5

Changing Cultures: Cultivate an Environment for a Professional Image

By Laura Cook Harrington, RN, MHA, CPHQ, CHCQM

Understanding Your Organization's Culture

As already discussed in the previous chapters, the image of nursing has changed dramatically through the past decades. From visual changes in our uniforms to changes in work demands, technology, training, and work ethics—all have influenced nursing's image and our professional culture.

But not all changes to our culture are imposed on us from outside forces. We can actively shape and improve our culture—whether it be the wider nursing image perceived by the public, or the professional culture on our unit. This chapter will help you evaluate and improve the culture at your organization.

Positive culture

All nurse managers want to work at an organization that has a positive, professional nursing culture: one that fosters respect and one where nurses are satisfied and engaged. But what is a professional culture? How does one cultivate a culture of excellence on one's unit? How do you measure your culture?

Creating a professional culture of excellence may seem overwhelming when you think about barriers, strategy, implementation, and the challenges you face within the dynamics of nursing. Why is it so difficult to instill a professional culture? The challenges vary within each organization, but there are many external and internal factors or barriers that influence a positive culture and therefore affect our ability to instill a professional nursing culture. The source of power and influence is you!

Determining culture

Your culture is the set of shared attitudes, values, goals, and practices that characterizes your unit or organization. Each nursing unit has its own culture, and the nursing department at your organization as a whole will also have a distinct culture.

It is a worthwhile endeavor for nurse leaders and unit-specific managers to take the time to define the current nursing culture within their organization. Identifying those things that affect the culture is important so that you understand any potential barriers to change. This will provide you with a wealth of knowledge about the current state of your culture and help you drive the things that you can change.

Requirements for culture change

Nursing culture is shaped by many internal factors, including barriers such as poor communication between leaders and frontline nurses or a lack of respect from medical staff. If nurses are not well respected by their colleagues on the medical staff, then how do you think you can create a culture of excellence?

Leadership plays a critical role in affecting culture throughout the organization. For example, imagine what happens if you have a manager who practices nothing but a punitive style of management, thus creating an environment in which the staff is scared to accept accountability and fears punishment. This would affect the unit's culture in many ways—none of them positive. Therefore, it is imperative that leadership stand behind nursing

and its vision to move toward a professional culture and a positive image of nursing. As a leader, it is important to create an environment for a culture that is professional, reaches for excellence, has mutual respect, and inspires values.

How Do We Change Culture?

This chapter will assist you in identifying barriers and then finding methods to implement positive cultural changes in your current structure by transforming it into a culture of excellence shared by all.

Step I: Define your current nursing culture (positives and negatives). What are the things that you like and dislike about the nursing culture in your organization? What are the things that you need to change? What are the barriers that will block change?

Step II: Identify the changes needed to enhance professional culture. Some changes take time, but there may be policies or changes in practice that can occur immediately. If you have a shared governance model with a "professional practice council," get that group to work on the strategy. For example, create a professional code of conduct and implement it immediately. Another policy that will drive professionalism is to create nursing expectations (see Figure 5.1 at the end of this chapter for an example). Remember: Once the policy is implemented, you must hold nurses accountable, or it is just another piece of paper that everyone ignores.

Don't forget to recognize and praise changes made throughout the year. Have you ever looked back and wondered, what did we accomplish this year? Keep a log of all the changes made in nursing for the year, and then communicate this to your nurses.

Step III: Create a nursing vision and mission

and then communicate this to the nursing staff. Creating a vision and mission will guide and provide structure for the nurses.

Step IV: Implement change that you can effect. Some changes will need to occur over many years, but these begin with the changes you can make now. Review the aspects of what you want to change, and then make it happen.

Resistance to change

Charles Dwyer stated, "Never expect anyone to engage in behavior that serves your values until you have given that person adequate reason to do so." Resistance to change comes in many different forms. For example, you may have a disruptive nurse or nurses acting unprofessionally and fighting within a unit. To create a professional culture, one step in this process would include creating a "nursing code of conduct." When implementing this you may get pushback, so the strategies to effect nursing change include:

- Establishing the need for change

- Having clear vision of your values

- Communicating the plan

- Identifying and dealing with the resistance

- Maintaining consistency and repeating the message

- Taking the heat from those resistant to change

- Dealing with unanticipated consequences

- Launching new initiatives

Major challenges in nursing today include apathy, lack of respect from colleagues, lack of professional identity, managing competing priorities (patient care versus other duties), physician-nurse communication, nurse-nurse relationships, team functioning, lack of critical-thinking skills, quality and patient safety, productivity, and others. It is important to identify and list the barriers to nursing excellence so that you can better understand what impacts your nursing culture.

Identify Levels of Organizational Change

When considering how to make changes in your organization, it's crucial to first understand the levels of organizational change.

Organizational change is twofold: revolutionary and evolutionary. Revolutionary changes are the major changes that affect deep structures; the type of changes where nothing will be the same again. Evolutionary changes are the type of changes where deep structure is not affected or greatly modified; about 95% of all organizational change falls into this evolutionary category. Therefore it will take some time to change culture—it is not simple and will not happen overnight. Nursing leaders—with administration's support—have to work together diligently to foster the right atmosphere and to promote a culture of excellence.

Change occurs at many levels of the organization:

- Individual

- Group or work unit

- Total organization

When reviewing organizational culture, you must break down specifically the level you are defining. For example, if you look at nursing, you can see the overall nursing culture, the specific cultures that exist within each unit (such as surgical services), and finally the organization's culture as a whole.

Think about your own organization and you can probably identify different cultures under one roof. For example, the medical staff probably has a different culture than nursing, each department or unit carries its own culture, and sometimes you may have distinct cultures on individual shifts. The inherent complexities of a hospital make it difficult for us to quickly move toward a positive culture. However, if nursing is unified and committed to making a change, it can be done.

When looking at the levels of organizational change, think about the barriers to change that exist and the way that change can be fostered at each of the three levels.

1. Individual

Individuals (you or your staff nurses) have their own values and beliefs. Each value or belief can be affected during the hiring and selection process, during working with others, in training and development, and through the pervasive unit culture. The cycle of staffing includes: recruitment and selection, training and development, coaching, and counseling.

Resistance to individual organizational change is due to the fear of losing something of value. Some techniques to use to overcome individual barriers to change are cited in the following table. The barriers include three different levels that affect the individual's behavior and how to overcome the barrier.

Barrier descriptor:	Blind
Behavior:	Intolerance to any change
Techniques to overcome barriers:	Provide reassurance; allow time to accept change
Barrier descriptor:	Political
Behavior:	Perception of value loss
Techniques to overcome barriers:	Provide reassurance; allow time to accept change
Barrier descriptor:	Ideological
Behavior:	Belief that change is wrong
Techniques to overcome barriers:	Counter with data and facts that change is positive

For example, some staff resist changes due to their ideological beliefs, and they view all change as negative. They resist change and put up resistance to change even though change is needed. To overcome this resistance and to encourage the individual to buy in to change, then you must provide data and facts to validate the change. For example, if all of a sudden nursing decided to change the procedures for caring for patients with diabetes, you might expect resistance from nurses who are used to providing care in a certain way. But if you include the evidence-based findings on nursing care for diabetic patients, then nurses have the data and facts that are needed for them to accept change. How can we expect nurses to accept change if we don't provide them with facts?

Another example is what happens when an organization makes changes to wage and benefit structure. Many nurses automatically assume the move is political and they perceive that management is changing the structure because it will be cheaper for the hospital. To gain trust and overcome pushback, the organization should lay out the benefits of the new wage and benefit structure compared to the old one.

2. Group or work unit

The second level of organizational change occurs at the group or work unit level, and group dynamics can be a major factor in influencing change. Group values and beliefs have significant effect on their members, and a group has more power than an individual.

Within this level there are three identified areas that play an important role in the group or work unit:

1. Team building

2. Self-directed

3. Intergroup

Further breakdown of these areas identifies the aspects of each level that must be addressed to change the group or work unit.

1. **Team building:**

- Set goals and priorities

- Analyze/allocate the way in which work is performed

- Examine the way the group is working (the process)

- Examine interpersonal relationships

2. **Self-directed:**

- Members learn to share power and leadership

- Effectively manage conflict

- Recognize differences in skills and abilities in deployment of human resources

3. **Intergroup:**

- Distinguish real conflict—there are substantive differences between personal conflict and the type of blaming behavior that can derive from mismanagement of agreement

- Develop effective methods of resolution

3. Total organization

The final level of change refers to change throughout the organization. Let's focus on nursing—instead of total organization—because it is where you have a span of control.

As identified above, it is essential for you to identify different nursing cultures throughout your organization, which includes reviewing individual, unit, and organizational levels. Looking at all three levels will provide you with the current cultural state and identify possible barriers to change at the individual, unit, or organizational level. Examining the nursing culture and making changes throughout the subsystems or units will help drive the desired change.

Lewin-Schein model of organizational change

The Lewin-Schein model of organizational change contains three stages:

- **Stage I is called unfreezing.** This is where you create motivation and readiness to change.

- **State II is called changing.** This is where you conduct the cognitive restructuring.

- **State III is called refreezing.** This is where you integrate the change fully into the culture to ensure the change is maintained.

This above model sums up a three-step process in driving cultural change that simplifies the complexity of accomplishing such tasks. Some nursing organizations have identified the urgent need within their structures to accept change. Some have begun to rebuild the structure through creating shared governance models that influence culture by giving nursing a voice. And some see this as impossible.

If we are going to define our legacy, what will it be? It is time for all of us to stand up for what we believe and make a positive impact on nursing. The impact we make today will ultimately impact patient care. This is what it is all about! This is why we must change a negative culture into a positive culture—for the sake of the patient.

Recognizing When We Have a Professional Nursing Culture

There are four components that identify a successful nursing organizational structure and foster a professional culture.

1. **Culture**

2. **Leadership**

3. **Structure and processes**

4. **Collaboration**

Each component adds value to the overall culture of nursing. So, in order for you to achieve excellence, you must have the following:

- **Culture** – A positive culture with effective communication and supportive relationships

- **Leadership** – Position descriptions, transformational leadership, novice-to-expert development and training, succession planning, selection, and rewards and recognition

- **Structure and processes** – Core competencies, nursing peer review, cultural diversity/competence, best practice protocols and acquiring and using data, policies/procedures, and credentialing

- **Collaboration** – Mutual support for strategic goals, collaborative relationships, mentorship, and nursing development planning

Each organization will have to determine what is important within the nursing structure. Once the components have been identified and you have identified the changes that must occur, then a plan can be developed.

It is advisable to develop indicators that will measure a professional culture of safety so that you can monitor ongoing performance. Some indicators that you are most likely reviewing now include: overall patient satisfaction with nursing care, safety indicators (including, but not limited to, falls), physician feedback on nursing care, etc. There are many types of indicators that help identify the performance of nursing. Other performance metrics might include: obtaining ANCC Magnet Recognition Program® designation, implementing a shared governance model, implementing nursing peer review, and so on. There is no end to the changes that can be made to better nursing and patient care.

Also, be aware of the challenges we all face when there are multiple levels of goals occurring at the same time. The board, administration, medical staff, departments, etc., all have goals, and sometimes it feels as though we are trying to cure world hunger when what we need to do is take a step back and identify the most important goals at the organizational level and nursing level. To be successful, it is important to create a plan that includes organizational goals and nursing goals. You probably have unit-level goals as well. Do not create a plan that is set up to fail because it is unattainable. You must make the complex simple, and that means focusing on what really matters.

In conclusion, you will know when you get there. The indicators will meet your benchmarks, there will be little nurse-to-nurse and physician-to-nurse conflict, physicians and patients will praise the nursing care, and there will be mutual collaboration and respect within the medical staff. With these in place, you will be able to sleep knowing that what you have accomplished has ultimately made a huge impact on patient care.

Clarifying expectations

Clarifying expectations can be a step toward defining the nurse culture in your work environment. Using the elements of Figure 5.1, work with other nurse leaders at your organization to develop consistent nurse practices. See Figure 5.1, which outlines nursing expectations.

FIGURE 5.1   NURSING EXPECTATIONS

The expectations described in this document reflect current nursing governance bylaws and hospital policies and procedures. This document is designed to bring together the most important issues found in those documents, along with some key concepts that reflect our nursing culture, vision, and standards of practice.

Nursing leaders will work to improve individual and aggregate nursing performance through nonpunitive approaches and appropriate positive and negative feedback. These strategies will allow each nurse the opportunity to grow and develop in his or her capabilities to provide outstanding patient care and make valuable contributions to our hospital and community.

Technical quality of care

- Achieve nursing outcomes that consistently meet or exceed generally accepted clinical standards for the nursing discipline
- Provide nursing care based upon the generally accepted clinical nursing standards and hospital policy
- Patient safety/patient rights
- Participate in hospital efforts to reduce adverse patient care events
- Protect patient information based on hospital policy/government regulations, and ensure that information is kept confidential
- Communicate all pertinent patient information to other members of the healthcare team
- Communicate effectively with patients and their families regarding nursing interventions and care
- Provide emotional and physical support to patients and families
- Provide comfort to patients, including prompt and effective nursing management
- Wear hospital identification at all times

Quality of service

- Provide timely and continuous nursing care to patients
- Maintain medical records consistent with the hospital policies, including, but not limited to, chart entry legibility and timely completion of initial nursing assessment, care plans, and notes
- When calling the attending physician, provide adequate communication regarding patient care needs, nursing interventions, and outcomes using the SBAR communication format:
  - Situation
  - Background
  - Assessment
  - Recommendation
- Support nursing leaders' and staff members' efforts to exceed patient satisfaction rates for nursing units

FIGURE 5.1   NURSING EXPECTATIONS (CONT.)

Resource utilization

- Strive to provide quality patient care that is cost-effective by cooperating with efforts to appropriately manage the use of valuable patient care resources
- Ensure patient care testing is scheduled when ordered and is timely
- Provide timely discharge instructions in collaboration with other caregivers

Peer and coworker relationships

- At all times act in a professional, respectful manner with patients, physicians, other nurses, administrators, board members, and other hospital personnel to enhance a spirit of cooperation and mutual respect and trust among members of the patient care team
- Refrain from inappropriate behavior as outlined in the "employee code of conduct" policy toward members of the hospital and medical staff, patients, or their families
- Refrain from documentation in the medical record that does not directly relate to the clinical status of the patient and plan of care or that is derogatory or inflammatory concerning the care provided to the patient

Contributions to hospital and community

- Participate, if requested, in relevant quality improvement activities or community services
- Support actions and decisions in accordance with the hospital's mission statement and strategic plan
- Review your individual and specialty data for all dimensions of performance, and utilize this data to continuously improve care

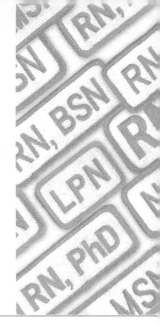

CHAPTER 6

Communication: Chiseling a New Image

By Kathleen Bartholomew, RN, MN

LEARNING OBJECTIVES

After reading this chapter, the participant will be able to:

✔ List reasons why nurses avoid communicating

✔ Explain how to use the DESC communication model

✔ Identify characteristics of professional communication

"Presidents like to think their administrations are based on big ideas, effective policies, and personal charm. But in a large part, the essential ingredient to their success is image—how they convey themselves to the public and how they communicate their goals to the country."

—*Kenneth T. Walsh*, U.S. News and World Report

How does nursing convey itself to the general public? As mentioned in previous chapters, the general public's image of today's nurse is "still largely inaccurate and negative. Nurses are underrepresented and often invisible in media portrayals of healthcare" (Kalisch, Begeny & Newman). The impact of the media on nursing's image has been profound. How nurses are portrayed in the media affects everything: recruitment, decision-making about policies concerning scope of practice and financing, and even consumer choices (Kalisch, Begeny & Newman).

The future of nursing is in jeopardy if we fail to communicate our goals to the country. In order for the nursing profession to do this, we must change the way we are accustomed to communicating with each other—especially when it comes to confrontation. This is where "the rubber meets the road," "the buck stops," and we "walk the talk"—or we don't.

Confrontation

Healthcare is characterized by a culture of silence, especially surrounding errors. Deeply embedded in both the physician and nurse culture is the belief that good nurses or good doctors don't make mistakes. Whether vocalized or not, we expect perfection from these human beings, and this unarticulated belief results in a culture of blame, shame, and most of all, silence. The statistics are illuminating:

- Seventy-eight percent of nurses said that it was difficult, if impossible, to confront a person or group directly (an example of keeping silent) if they exhibited incompetent care

- Eighty-eight percent of MDs say they work with people who show poor clinical judgment

- Fewer than 10% of MDs, RNs, and clinical staff directly confront their colleagues about concerns

(Source: "Silence Kills: The Seven Crucial Conversations for Healthcare" study by VitalSmarts. Available at *www.silencekills.com.*)

This inability to speak is called "self-silencing." The term was coined in 1991 by Jack, who found that people silence themselves because they value the relationship above anything else. Yet communication errors cause more accidental deaths than any other type of error. The fact that we are not

talking becomes more than a cultural shift: it is our ethical and moral obligation to create a communication culture where we can say everything that is on our minds at all times.

> *"One day in surgery a 17-year-old coded. The anesthesiologist had accidentally selected a vial of epinephrine instead of the intended 10 mg of Toradol. A root-cause analysis revealed that the doctor was distracted—talking on his cell phone to his stockbroker while administering the medicine. As part of the investigation team, my first question to the OR nurses was, "What if that was your 17-year-old boy on the table? Would you have said something then?"*

The reality is that the most common confrontation style nurses use is avoidance. Nurses frequently demonstrate a passive-aggressive style of communicating (meaning, they will tell everyone on the unit why they are upset with you, but they won't actually come and talk to you themselves). This behavior was role-modeled and then adopted by generation after generation of nurses who grew up in a male-dominated culture. Now, however, we have both an opportunity and responsibility to affect nursing's image. And this incredible profession now needs every single nurse's immediate support and protection. Learning how to confront each other is critical to patient safety, our image, and our future.

"Our lives begin to end the day we become silent about things that matter"

—*M. L. King*

Having a crucial conversation

There are steps you can take to become more comfortable and more adept at confronting other people:

- Think of a conversation that you want to have at your workplace—the one you've been putting off. Imagine that someone has assured you that it will turn out okay.

- Who do you need to talk to? What about?

- Now, rate how painful it will be for you to have this conversation on the pain scale of 1–10. Pick the very first number that comes to your mind.

- Stop for a moment and identify the reason that you are not engaging in this particular conversation.

Why aren't nurses having these conversations? Nearly one thousand nurses have shared their thought process as I have asked this question in workshops across the country, and as it turns out, there are a lot of similarities. The key reasons are:

- Fear of retaliation

- Fear of being labeled

- Fear of rejection

- Fear of the outcome

- Fear of being fired

- Fear of being misunderstood

- Fear of failure

- Fear of making the relationship worse or putting it in jeopardy

Fear is the common denominator in all of these answers. Our silence is a result of these fears. *This silence is a critical factor in our invisibility.* As a profession, we are not engaging in the crucial conversations necessary to build self and group esteem. Why? Because we underestimate the effect of culture and history on our everyday conversations.

The foundation of all communication is who you are. In every single conversation you have, whether conscious or not, you make a decision. How much risk am I willing to take? How much of my authentic self will I reveal? In the past, to be so vulnerable resulted in harm or a poor outcome for many of us, so we hesitate to venture into that authentic place again. Without even realizing it, we surrender to every human being's greatest needs: safety and belonging.

As it turns out, to be accepted by a group is a critical and basic need of all human beings—and one of the easiest ways to be accepted by any group is to emulate their behavior. Only when nurses summon the courage and develop the skill set to start taking conversational risks will the image of nursing change. First, we elevate ourselves in each other's eyes, and then in the public's eyes. What is required is to be yourself (flaws and all) while holding yourself and others accountable. Communication is the tool, the chisel by which we will shape our new image. There is nothing more powerful than not being afraid; nothing more effective than speaking your truth at all times; and nothing that will help nursing more than increasing our ability to have meaningful dialogues with each other.

The Skill Set: Tell Me How

A steady gaze, a firm handshake, and a pleasant, confident tone are all critical factors in communication, but the most important factors are:

1. Your willingness to not judge others until you have heard their stories

2. Your ability to speak your truth about your own story

You don't have to be right or prove someone else wrong, just willing to "come to the table" and speak to the person or situation you are concerned about. Then, one of the most difficult hurdles becomes simply knowing how or where to begin.

One comment I receive all the time is "I just don't know where to start." This is where the DESC communication model is very helpful.

Also take a look at Figure 6.1 for further information on how to use the DESC tool.

DESC COMMUNICATION MODEL

D – Describe the behavior

E – Explain the effect of the behavior

S – State the desired outcome

C – Consequence: Say what will happen if the behavior continues

(Source: Sharon Cox, MSN, RN, CNAA. Cox & Associates)

Some people prefer to memorize the key words that represent this model because it gives them a consistent structure to follow:

D When . . .

E I feel . . . because . . .

S Therefore, I want/need . . .

C So that . . .

DESC COMMUNICATION MODEL EXAMPLES

Take a look at the model in action in the following situations.

Example: You walk into a patient's room and the patient reports poor nursing care—she hasn't had a bath in two days. Now you need to talk to the day nurse who was responsible for that patient. Where do you start? With the only thing you know. Be specific and stick to the facts. Monitor your own feelings about the situation because they will come out in your tone of voice or other nonverbal cues.

D   Describe. *"Tammy, can I talk to you for a moment in private? I just came out of room 942 and Mrs. Wiggins told me that she hasn't had a bath for the last two days."*

E   Explain the effect of the behavior. *"I'm concerned about this patient's report, as the standard of care here is for patients to receive a daily bath."*

PAUSE, PAUSE, PAUSE.

This PAUSE provides a space for the other person to take in the information and respond. There may be no further words needed. In this case, the nursing assistant recalled that the patient was so nauseated the first postop day that she refused a bath, and the second postop day an occupational therapist (OT) was walking the patient to the bathroom and the OT said she would put the patient in the shower.

The nurse responded: *"Thank you for bringing this to my attention. Next time someone promises to do a job that I am responsible for, I will remember to check back and make sure that it was done."*

Sometimes, conversations are a little more difficult. They are rated higher on our conversational pain scale. After we pause, there is silence. How do you keep the conversation going and arrive at a place of understanding?

Example: I work with someone who is always making negative comments. What can I say?

D   Describe: *"Can I talk to you for a moment in private? When you came on to the floor at the beginning of the shift and found out that it was your turn to float, I heard you make some really negative comments. The same thing happened yesterday and last Monday."*

E   Explain: *"I understand that everyone has bad days, but I need you to know that your comments really depress me. They bring me down."*

S   State what you need: *"I need you to know and understand that your comments have a big influence on my mood—and I can see them affecting others as well."*

C   Consequence: *"If I have to continue to listen to this, I am concerned that this negativity will affect my morale and health, as well as our relationship and others on the team."*

FIGURE 6.1 A CLOSER LOOK AT DESC

Feedback Formula	Rationale	DESC Model (Intent/impact)	Rationale
Facts first	Lead with the facts! Observable, less likely to cause defensiveness, facts are not personal. Facts are seen and heard. Verifiable by others.	Describe the situation.	Describe using facts, orient the person to the issue you are discussing with them.
Story second	Your story is your impression, your interpretation of the facts. Share what the facts meant to you. Your story usually has some emotion attached to it, the facts have caused you to "feel" something. Share your story.	Explain what this means to you.	Let the person know the impact of the situation. Tell them how you "see it." This tells them why you are talking to them . . . it is having an impact on you. Share that.
Pause, pause, pause	Pausing allows the other person a minute to assimilate what they have just heard. It also prevents you from overwhelming the person and from speaking too fast.	Pause, pause, pause	Pausing allows the other person a minute to assimilate what they have just heard. It also prevents you from overwhelming the person and speaking too fast.
Check for understanding	Asking, *"How do you see it?"* or *"Do you see it differently?"* invites dialogue. This step is about clarifying the situation you are giving feedback about.	State what you want instead.	Discuss behavior you DO want. Be descriptive. Using the affirmative approach helps the other person know what they should do and minimizes defensiveness by not focusing on what is wrong. This step reframes the situation: "This is what I do want from you." The positive approach can make it easier for the other person to agree with you. It helps them save face.
		Consequences: describe the consequences that will naturally occur if the situation continues. (Motivation is different for each person. Try to describe consequences that matter to this person.)	Describe the impact if the person does not meet the expectation you just "stated." Consequences usually have an impact on three levels: **Individual:** *"What is in it for me?"* What pain or pleasure is attached to this situation? Outline the benefit to them associated with complying. **Social:** Impact to others, to the team. What praise or pressure from others might be a consequence? **Work environment:** Standards, policies, rules, *"carrots and sticks"* associated with this situation. Progressive Corrective Action is an example of a work consequence/impact.

Source: Adapted from Sharon Cox's DESC model. Courtesy of Anastasia Hartog, Employee Learning, Swedish Medical Center, Seattle.

Professional Communication

Every interaction that we have with another person at work is a communication. Even if we never speak at all, our body language communicates whether we are interested or disengaged, caring or aloof. More than anything, we communicate what we think of ourselves. The image that we project to others is exactly how we feel. If we feel like a long-suffering martyr for healthcare, this image comes through. If we feel like a skilled expert who can compassionately deliver excellent patient care, everyone who comes within five feet of us knows it without us ever saying a word.

Sometimes, however, we run into communication that is not always professional. The basis of professional communication is respect. People who consider themselves professionals (lawyers, judges, physicians, etc.) adhere to a set of standards that are different from those who act unprofessionally. It's the difference between people who see themselves as powerless, and people who are empowered.

The following behaviors are characteristics of professionals:

- Always stop and look people in the eye when you are speaking to them

- Never stand by listening while one coworker puts down another

- Never criticize in public; always ask to speak to the person directly in private

- Keep confidences

- Work cooperatively, despite feelings of dislike

- Be willing to help when help is requested (or you notice a coworker overwhelmed)

- Don't participate in gossip

- Stand up for the absent member in a conversation

- Respect the privacy of others

- Address coworkers by their first names, and ask for help and advice when needed

Source: Adapted from Arglye & Henderson, 1985; Chasta, 2001. SLACK Incorporated and The Journal of Continuing Education in Nursing.

> At first, Mandy didn't know what to do and she felt helpless. The staffing levels on the floor were horrible and for months staff had been complaining to her as the charge nurse. Morale was terrible. She had already gone to the manager three times and now staff members are talking about quitting. Mandy went to the manager's office yet again, but this time with a plan.
>
> *"I know that I've come to you several times about the staffing issues and you've said you can't do anything about it. I am now ready to bring this up to a higher level. I've made an appointment with the CNO and I wanted you to know because I would appreciate your support if you can come."*

Dealing with Unprofessional Coworkers

As you are picking up your assignment for the shift, you notice someone rolling his or her eyes, followed by a quick darting glance toward you. Or as you walk into the nurses' lounge, you hear the tail end of a conversation about how you dump on the next shift. Or perhaps you hear a rumor circulating about the *real* reason why you are no longer precepting. How does a professional handle unprofessional behaviors? And how does a professional respond to nonverbal communication?

Unprofessional behaviors between peers fall into the category of horizontal hostility. These are the overt and covert ways that people put each other down: from eye-rolling and silence to backstabbing and gossip. Sociologists have found that when a group of people feel like they have no power, they start lashing out at each other. Fortunately, everyone in the group has the opportunity to change the group dynamics as, one by one, they start realizing the tremendous impact of their behavior on each other.

UNPROFESSIONAL BEHAVIORS

When you see any of the following behaviors, a conversation is no longer optional.

OVERT Name-calling, bickering, fault-finding, backstabbing, criticism, intimidation, gossip, shouting, blaming, using put-downs, raising eyebrows, etc.

COVERT Unfair assignments, silence, eye-rolling, ignoring, refusal to work with someone, sabotage, isolation, sighing, whining, fabrication, etc.

- Don't wait—the sooner you confront the behavior, the better.

- Always ask to speak to the person in private.

- Take a few deep, centering breaths before you begin the conversation.

- If you are sitting down, sit at right angles instead of across from each other. (If you rate this conversation a 9 or 10 on our conversation pain scale, don't sit at all; instead, go for a walk.)

- Remember the goal: Speak your truth. (You can't make people change, but when you speak your truth, people can see the impact, and another's behavior change is more likely to happen.)

- Remember: When someone is loud, aggressive, or mean, they are angry or afraid (and anger is a secondary emotion; try to get to the primary emotion, which is hurt).

- Whenever you don't know what to do, repeat what the other person said: "Let me get this straight. You are saying that...."

 The Image of Nursing

Unprofessional Physicians

We work with physicians more frequently than with any other member of the healthcare team. Sometimes, we experience unprofessional behaviors from physicians as well. How do you know when it is important to have a conversation with a physician? A conversation is mandatory any time anyone makes you feel less than the competent caregiver you are.

Physician behaviors also fall into the categories of overt or covert:

Overt: Raised voice or yelling, fault-finding, criticism, intimidation, hanging up/slamming the phone, throwing a chart/instrument, etc.

Covert: Never bothering to learn your name, ignoring you or your comments, refusing to listen, poor or absent eye contact, etc.

Just as nurses have passed on behaviors through generations, so have physicians. The key to healthy physician-nurse communication is truly understanding that these unprofessional behaviors are *learned behaviors* and that the physician will remain unaware of the impact of these behaviors *unless you say something*. Unprofessional physician behaviors immobilize us because we take then personally. The key with physicians is to begin every crucial conversation with the words, "May I speak to you for a moment in private?" The practice of taking someone aside to speak to them about important matters is an integral part of the physician culture, and physicians will always say yes. Then, use the DESC model you learned—or your own voice.

Whenever you are communicating with a level above in the hierarchy—manager, physician, administration—it takes more courage than usual. But the results are well worth the risk because the damage to your self-esteem if you don't say something is far more destructive.

Cary had worked night shift for over five years. One physician's tone of voice was particularly degrading when she (or anyone else) needed to call him. One night she called for some pain medication and was treated extremely rudely. The next morning, Cary met the doctor in the hall:

"May I speak to you for a moment in private?" she asked.

The physician nodded and they stepped aside. *"First of all,"* she said, *"I called you in the middle of the night because you were the physician on call and your patient was hurting badly. I needed an order for pain medication. And secondly, I didn't appreciate the way you treated me on the phone—as if I just thought up something I needed to bother you with, like a stool softener. This was a much needed medication and I would appreciate it in the future if you would not use the demeaning, angry tone of voice you did last night."*

Rehema knew Dr. Barton was in a hurry because the first surgery had taken over an hour longer than expected. Then, at the second surgery, the patient had a bleed that was difficult to stop. By the time they opened the third case, Dr. Barton was livid—rudely shouting orders to everyone, including her, in the room. Rehema waited until the next day before approaching the physician with her concerns. "Dr. Barton," she said, hesitating for just a moment. *"I'd like to speak to you in private for a moment about something that is causing me great concern."*

Difficult Patients

Another challenge to nurses can be the patients themselves. When scared, hurt, angry, or confused, patients can exhibit extremely rude behaviors. Once again, realize that this is not directed at you personally and always maintain your professional decorum. From my experience, nurses handle these situations very well—in the room. But when they go out to the nurses' station, they vent and start talking about the patient. Professionals do not gossip or create a scene for moral support at the expense of the privacy of the patient. If you need to vent, take the charge nurse aside and share your frustration while gaining support and understanding in private.

In addition, don't ever be a silent witness and stand by and listen as another nurse is slamming a physician, peer, or patient.

DESC COMMUNICATION MODEL EXAMPLES FOR COVERT BEHAVIORS

Example 1: What do you say after you hear a rumor that a coworker has been backstabbing you?

D *"I'd like to talk with you in private. I heard from another nurse that you said I didn't know what I was doing, and that I would never be a good nurse."*

E *"When I hear that someone has been saying things about me and I don't know why, or even what situation it pertains to, I feel sabotaged and set up to fail."*

S *"I want to be a good nurse and I can't do that without your honest feedback and support. Can you say what you feel and think directly to me and in private?"*

C *"Without your support, I am sure to fail. I will have to find another place to work even though I like this specialty."*

Example 2: How do I communicate with my manager about unprofessional behaviors on the unit without sounding like I am complaining or putting other nurses down?

D *"I'd like to speak with you about the culture of blame surrounding mistakes on the unit. I am hearing a lot of indirect conversation going on about errors. On several occasions, when a nurse from the previous shift has made a mistake, it is whispered to everyone else on the next shift."*

E *"This gossip makes me hyper-vigilant and sets up other nurses on the unit for scapegoating. It is decreasing my morale and self-esteem."*

S *"I need this to stop."*

C *"I cannot work in an environment where anything less than perfection is ridiculed and where we ignore the fact that we are human and need to openly discuss errors as learning experiences."*

Can you feel the difference as you read these examples? What words would you use to describe these conversations? They are positive, supportive responses filled with integrity and spoken by people who truly value themselves. Despite the unprofessional situation, these are professionals who have used their conversations to rise to and maintain a level of professionalism.

 The Image of Nursing

Responding to Nonverbal Communication

The biggest problem that nurses say they encounter is nonverbal communication or innuendos. Covert behaviors increase our stress level because the situation is ambiguous, and researchers have found that uncertainty increases stress. Did the charge nurse intend to make out an unfair assignment, or was she truly unaware of the acuity of the patients? Did your peer refuse to help you last shift, or did she really not see you were drowning?

Only 7% of communication is verbal, which means the overwhelming majority of communication is nonverbal. Our bodies are constantly saying what our minds are thinking—whether we are aware of these thoughts or not. That's why when we approach someone about an error, it goes all wrong, because the recipient is already picking up on the feeling that we think it's their fault, or they're inadequate, or we are angry. Whether dealing with overt or covert messages, the DESC model will provide you with an excellent framework.

TIP

Take the conversation you identified earlier (the one you should be having but are not) and apply the DESC model. Imagine going to this person and having the conversation turn out very well. Now, make it a reality.

"Time is not a line, but a series of now points." —Taisen Deshimaru

Life is not a line, but a series of points *because any point can change the direction of the line.* What is the point where nursing's image will change? What is the point where we will be esteemed by our peers, honored by society, and known by our patients, who will understand our true role in providing safe, quality care? How can we change the direction of the line and point it toward a new image of a professional nurse?

Chiseling a New Image

The hope of our profession is in your very next interaction or communication with your peers, the very next opportunity that you have to make a decision: to speak or be silent; to be passive or assertive; hostile or supportive; aware or oblivious.

These are the pivotal moments that will propel nursing into a positive new image. There will be no edict from above, and no mandate from administration, the government, or a nursing organization that will change the course for us. Rather, the elevation of our profession will come from within as, one by one, we raise our awareness, speak our truth, value ourselves and our work, and discover our greatest strengths in each other.

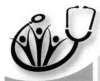

Personal Perspectives: Recently Graduated Nurse

By Tanya Becks, RN

Making the transition from student to RN

As a student nurse, I wanted to get the most that I possibly could out of my education and time as a student. I went to all my classes, I studied, and I worked for the good grades that I got. I also got involved with other students in group projects, and I tutored lower-level courses in nursing, as well as the life science courses (prerequisite classes for the nursing program). I went to my clinicals with the attitude that I was there to learn all I could and do the work to the best of my ability, so that when I was done with nursing school, I would be as prepared as possible. While I was in class and at clinicals, I always tried to glean as much information as possible from peers, instructors, and most importantly the nurses we were working with, to help make the transition from student to working nurse as smooth as possible. Most of the people I talked to said it usually takes a year of working to feel like you are "getting it." Another good piece of advice I got from the seasoned nurses is that one never knows everything. There is always something new to learn, whether it is a new way to do something, a new procedure, a new disease process, or a new medication.

I think it has been beneficial to me to realize that it will take a while to truly get into my groove of being a nurse. I worked hard through nursing school and was involved in leadership, student life, and the overall academia. And I will continue to work hard as a new nurse. Transitioning from my role as a student to a working nurse in these areas is a continuing process. I didn't learn everything I needed while I was in school, so I will continue to learn. I have joined a team of nurses at a local hospital, and already I am feeling like we are a family of sorts. This "family" feeling is important in our field—we need to be able to have an older and more experienced "sibling" who we can go to when we new nurses have questions and need help.

I think that the leadership aspect of transition is the most difficult to conceptualize. I certainly do not want to appear bossy or like a know-it-all, but I think that as nurses we are all leaders—not necessarily of each other, but leaders in the healthcare profession as we take care of our patients. It is important to be confident in our work, to prioritize, and to delegate when appropriate. A good leader works as a team player, not as a dictator. I also think that the leadership aspect can be applied to how we as nurses—both seasoned and new—treat the future nurses, the student nurses that we work with from time to time. It is important to make them feel like they are part of our team, rather than someone who is just fumbling and in our way as we rush from one patient to another.

NURSING VOICES

A good leader is a role model who doesn't burn bridges. I think this is one area of nursing that needs improvement, but as more nurses view themselves as leaders, the image of nursing will improve and strengthen.

Tanya Becks is a registered nurse currently working and residing in Michigan. As a student nurse at Lansing Community College, she traveled to Africa to perform cardiovascular screenings in a village in Ghana. She is pursuing graduate studies with an emphasis on natural therapies and community health. She is interested in travel nursing, and would be especially interested in becoming a nurse for a circus.

REFERENCES

Bartholomew, K. (2007). *Stressed Out About Communication Skills.* Marblehead, MA: HCPro, Inc.

Bartholomew, K. (2006). *Ending Nurse-to-Nurse Hostility: Why Nurses Eat Their Young and Each Other.* Marblehead, MA: HCPro, Inc.

Bartholomew, K. (2004). *Speak Your Truth: Proven Strategies for Effective Nurse-Physician Communication.* Marblehead, MA: HCPro, Inc.

Jack, Dana Crowley. (1991). *Silencing the Self: Women and Depression.* New York: HarperCollins.

Kalisch, B., Begeny, S., and Newmann, S. (2007). "The image of the nurse on the Internet." *Nursing Outlook* 55 (4):182–188.

VitalSmarts. (2008). "Silence Kills: The Seven Crucial Conversations for Healthcare." Available at *www.silencekills.com.*

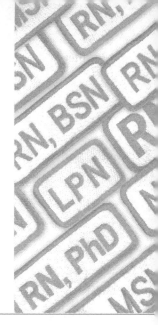

CHAPTER 7

Nursing Image and the ANCC Magnet Recognition Program®

By Barbara J. Hannon, RN, MSN, CPHQ

LEARNING OBJECTIVES

After reading this chapter, the participant will be able to:

✔ Identify the Force of Magnetism related to nursing image

✔ Discuss the role of nursing image in the ANCC Magnet Recognition Program®

✔ Recognize strategies used by designated organizations to promote nursing staff

As Karen Tomajan discussed in Chapter 3, images of nurses, in both print and electronic media, have created powerful pictures in the minds of the public, patients, and nurses themselves. Many of these images are negative and exploitative, but they have nonetheless left a mark on the public, leading to confusion over who nurses are and what they do.

The lack of a consistently positive nursing image is exacerbating the nursing shortage. As baby boomer nurses retire and leave the profession, we are facing a critical shortfall of nurses in the coming decades, and recruitment of new generations of nurses is crucial. Therefore, the importance of defining, maintaining, and supporting a positive, consistent image of nurses needs to be a priority.

For the profession to recruit and retain bright young nurses, the image of the profession needs to be defined by nurses themselves in a consistently positive light that shows nurses positioned to affect healthcare delivery through excellence in education, research, quality management, and collaborative practice. To do this, nurses themselves need to take charge of their own image.

Formal Recognition

The American Nurses Credentialing Center (ANCC) Magnet Recognition Program® (MRP) is a powerful ally in defining and promoting a positive image of nurses and is a program developed by nurses and for nurses. Through the designation process, hospitals achieve a level of public recognition that elevates nurses to the forefront of patient care excellence and highlights nurses' contributions to healthcare to the public, insurers, quality forums, patients, and other healthcare providers.

Hospitals that aspire to MRP designation must weave a picture of their nurses as integral to the success of the hospital and vital to the success of patient outcomes. Nurses in MRP hospitals must be seen by the public, their communities, governing boards, physicians, and other healthcare providers as essential components of successful patient care environments.

Nursing image is woven through all the components of the MRP program and aspiring hospitals must show evidence that nurses are at the forefront of patient care, using quality improvement processes, evidence-based practice, scientific inquiry, and critical thinking to improve patient care and safety.

In fact, one of the Forces of Magnetism—the essential components or attributes of the MRP program that demonstrate excellence—is solely related to the image of nursing at the organization. Force 12: Image of Nursing falls under the second model component—Structural Empowerment—in the 2008 revisions to the program. Placing nursing image under the concept of "empowerment" ensures that nurses themselves take responsibility for promoting a positive image of nursing.

The MRP demands that nurses at all levels contribute to patient excellence, strategic planning, and organizational policies, and that nurses are recognized in multiple ways by the institution for their contributions. Organizations must provide evidence of contributions by bedside, direct care nurses in multiple sources of evidence in the application documents.

Image Takes Center Stage

The Force of Magnetism on image of nursing requires hospitals show that "Nurses are viewed as integral to the organization's ability to provide patient care services and that the services provided by nurses are characterized as essential by other members of the organization" (ANCC 2005).

In today's healthcare environment, nurses provide approximately 90% of bedside patient care, putting the nursing profession in a prime position to influence patient outcomes. To ensure organizational success, nurses need to be involved in the development of strategic priorities and aligned with the direction of their institution. In addition, because nurses comprise the largest work force within acute-care institutions, recognition for their contributions must pervade the institution and be demonstrated in marketing and publications, as well as within the halls of the organization for public display. Force of Magnetism 12 requires nursing departments and hospitals to show evidence of how nurses are valued, respected, and recognized in multiple ways by the organization and community.

Influence of the chief nursing officer

In addition to the definition of nursing image, the program also identifies two important components to the force. The first relates to the influence the chief nursing officer (CNO) exerts on organizational strategic planning and decision-making at the highest level of institutional leadership. As the head of the nursing department, the CNO must sit at the table with all senior management and influences the direction of the entire organization—not just the direction of the nursing department. The CNO sets the standard for nurses in the institution.

The way in which institutional leadership perceives the entire nursing staff is likely based on senior leadership's perception of the CNO. In MRP designated organizations, the CNO is involved in high-level decisions including capital budget determination, committee searches for department heads, personnel policies, interdisciplinary planning, and strategic planning. CNOs are also viewed by organizational stakeholders as having equal status with other senior decision-makers.

Perception of nursing

The second component concerns how all levels of nurses are perceived throughout the organization not only by other disciplines, but by the organization's leadership, the community, and by nurses themselves. In MRP environments, nurses must be viewed as essential for excellence in patient outcomes and to the success of the institution.

Research indicates that recognition of nursing's accomplishments by organizations contributes to nurses' overall satisfaction with their jobs. In MRP organizations, nurses at all levels and across all departments are perceived as professionals who are essential to the provision of quality healthcare and integral to the success of the organization. The perception that nurses are the institution's keys to influencing outcomes must be demonstrated by clear evidence from nonnursing organizational leadership, employees from other disciplines, patients and nurses, and the community served by the facility.

Strategies to Promote Nursing Image

Designated organizations—or those on the MRP journey—often pursue numerous strategies to improve and showcase a positive image of nursing, and these strategies can be used by any organization wanting to celebrate its nurses.

Nurse leaders can develop a marketing plan to portray their nurses in a positive way, and organizations can use marketing and media experts to help them develop professional recruitment literature or promotional advertising and to help them develop external media contacts. Organizational and departmental internal and external Web sites can be used to portray a positive image and celebrate the organization's nurses. Units can use display cabinets, posters, and pictures to portray nursing accomplishments. Print media—including pamphlets, newsletters, annual reports, magazines, and other publications, whether departmental or organizationwide—can be used to demonstrate positive images of nursing and the collaboration between nursing and community organizations can be used to promote nurses and the profession of nursing outside of the organization.

Published leadership profiles

Many organizations publish leadership profiles in both electronic and print media. These profiles include the CNO and other high-level nursing leaders. In addition, many institutions have portraits of hospital leaders mounted on walls in key areas of the hospital. The CNO should be pictured alongside other senior leaders, as befits the status of the organization's nursing department executive.

Internal and external Web sites

External Web sites are one of the most popular ways of marketing healthcare organizations. These organizational Web sites profile the department of nursing, nursing leaders, nursing accomplishments, and newsworthy items involving nurses. External Web sites contain simple links for viewers to connect to the nursing department external Web site, where the majority of positive nursing information can be found by patients, clients, families, and prospective nurse employees. Take advantage of today's technology by featuring streaming videos of nurses, interviews with hospital nurses, and links to newsworthy events. Such Web sites can be a powerful tool in showcasing a professional department of nursing.

Internal Web sites (or intranets) are another powerful tool, where nurses within the organization can find and post information about their colleagues. Intranets can be used to display awards, recognitions, publications, and profiles of staff. They can highlight little-known nontraditional roles such as informatics nurses, professional development nurses, or nurse researchers, and can be used to show the positive effect these nontraditional roles can have on the image of nursing within the organization.

Newsletters

Most organizations publish newsletters with information about the hospital. Organizational newsletters can include sections on nurse accomplishments, and the department of nursing should be vigilant that each issue provides a positive view of the organization's nurse accomplishments.

Many departments of nursing also publish nursing newsletters. These include notable nurse accomplishments and profiles of staff nurses. They can also be used to discuss nurses' attendance at conferences and any poster presentations or publications by the organization's nurses.

Many patient care units also publish their own unit newsletters. Desktop publishing software makes such newsletters easy to produce, and they provide a positive image of nurses at the bedside level. These newsletters should be posted where patients, families, and other healthcare providers can read them and see that unit's accomplishments.

Annual reports

Most hospitals publish annual reports of the organization listing accomplishments of the institution over the previous year. Departments of nursing need to be vigilant that these reports include profiles of nursing accomplishments alongside the accomplishments of physicians and other disciplines in the organization.

Local media

Nurses can find the local media to be their allies in promoting a positive image. Developing a relationship with these groups will allow you to alert them to nursing accomplishments, which they can use in their respective mediums. This can be done through a marketing representative, the MRP project director, or another nurse leader who can feed interesting stories to print or television reporters. Items that local media may consider publishing include nursing research projects, awards, or human interest stories involving nurses and patients.

REFERENCES

American Nurses Credentialing Center (2005). *The Magnet Recognition Program: Recognizing Excellence in Nursing Service Application Manual.* Silver Spring, MD: ANCC.

Cole, R.C. (2001). "Magnet hospitals use culture, not wages, to solve the nursing shortage." *Journal of Healthcare Management* 46 (4): 224–227.

Hallam, J. (2000). *Nursing the Image: Media, Culture and Professional Identity.* London: Routledge.

Jones, A. (1989). *Images of Nurses: Perspective from History, Art and Literature.* Philadelphia: University of Pennsylvania Press.

Reverby, S. (1987). *Ordered to Care: The Dilemma of American Nursing 1850 to 1945.* New York: Cambridge University Press.

Sigma Theta Tau International and the University of Rochester School of Nursing. (1997). Woodhull Study on Nursing and the Media. Available at *www.nursingsociety.org.*

Vanderbilt University Medical Center School of Nursing and Center for Healthcare Services. February 2004. "Vanderbilt Nursing Survey." Available at *www.nurseweek.com.*

Finding Our Voice: An Image of Professionalism and Nursing Excellence

By Diana Swihart, PhD, DMin, MSN, CS, RN-BC

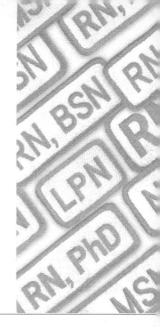

After reading this chapter, the participant will be able to:

✔ List criteria for judging nursing excellence

✔ Discuss ways managers can encourage staff to strive for professional excellence

"Excellence is an art won by training and habituation. We do not act rightly because we have virtue or excellence, but we rather have those because we have acted rightly. We are what we repeatedly do. Excellence, then, is not an act but a habit." – Aristotle

The Profession of Nursing

Florence Nightingale established the first nursing school to give nurses a voice that would eventually be heard globally and across generations. She insisted on curriculum to educate nurses who would act intelligently while remaining committed to serving others through evidence-based professional nursing care (Nightingale, 1859). Prior to Nightingale's reforms, a doctor of the 1800s described nurses of that time as "dull, unobservant, untaught women; of the best it could only be said that they were kindly and careful and attentive in doing what they were told" (quoted in Schuyler 1992).

Today professional nurses from all academic levels and practice settings work collaboratively with physicians and other healthcare providers to effect the best possible patient outcomes. Although nurses still embody the characteristics of compassionate care, they have become scientists, researchers, administrators, and direct care providers with their own advances in knowledge and acquired skills.

Guanci describes a combination of tenets (2007) that reflects elements of Miller's "Wheel of Professionalism" (Chitty & Black, 2007) and represents professional nursing practice as an intellectual discipline separate from other professions, such as medicine or education. Nursing as a profession encompasses:

- A well-defined body of knowledge

- Depth of education

- Control over nursing practice and the practice environment

- Self-regulation

- Use of evidence-based practice and nursing research

- Peer review

- The ability to practice autonomously

- Affiliation with professional organizations

- A system of values

- The development of a unique relationship with the patient

In many ways, though, the image of nurses still resonates with the 1800s description.

The general public does not see or understand to what degree nurses affect their care and well-being. They do not think of nurses as *professionals*. Buresh and Gordon (2006) emphasize the disparity between what nurses do and what others (non-nurses) *think* nurses do. This is our failure, one from which we must move forward if we are ever to experience genuine nursing excellence, collaborative partnerships, and public recognition of nursing as a valued profession.

But what is *nursing excellence*? *Excellence* means rising above the mediocrity of "business as usual" and redefining the boundaries of success. *Nursing excellence is grounded in professionalism and built on relationships that challenge us to reach new heights of engagement and risk. It is measured in outcomes related to practice, quality, and competency (Koloroutis 2004). Martin Luther King Jr. captured the essence of nursing excellence when he said, "All labor that uplifts humanity has dignity and importance and should be undertaken with painstaking excellence."

Defining Excellence

What, then, does *nursing excellence* actually look like? Many agencies and organizations have established criteria to signify excellence, such as the Malcolm Baldrige National Quality Program, The Joint Commission, and the American Nurses Credentialing Center's (ANCC's) Magnet Recognition Program® (McClure & Hinshaw 2002). Although they differ in specifics, they offer the same general qualities as sources of evidence for excellence in healthcare. The following represent some of the essentials of a culture of *nursing* excellence:

- Staff-centered, patient-focused, servant leadership in all levels of administration and executive commitment

- Nurses are represented on interprofessional and interdisciplinary teams and committees (e.g., strategic planning teams, hospital ethics committee)

- Exemplary patient, nurse, and physician satisfaction surveys

- Collaborative and collegial nurse/physician relationships

- Learning environments that support nurses academically and through continuing education and specialty certification

- Nurses belong to professional organizations

- Professional competency and commitment to continual quality improvement

- Continuous improvements in productivity and patient flow rates

- Nurse-sensitive quality indicators exceeding national benchmarks and internal performance measures

- Nurse responsibility, accountability, and autonomy in all practice settings

- Direct care nurses engage in nursing research at the bedside

- Evidence-based practice is reflected in patient care structures, processes, and outcomes

- Retention over time of educated and experienced direct care nurses and nurse leaders

The ANCC Magnet Recognition Program® (MRP) designation is currently the highest validation of professional nursing excellence that an organization can attain. MRP organizations are globally respected for the knowledge and expertise of their nurses. (American Nurses Credentialing Center 2005).

These are the leaders in nursing excellence, restructuring the image of nursing into one of healthcare reformation; discovery through nursing research; and innovation in the delivery of care for patients, families, and communities.

Improving the Image of Nurse Professionalism and Excellence

How can we improve the image of nursing professionalism and excellence? Try the following exercises and clinical applications and find out for yourself!

To make professionalism and excellence in nursing a habit and not just an occasional act, as Aristotle cautioned, do as many of the following as you can, today and throughout your career:

- Explore the American Nurses Credentialing Center's Web site at *www.nursecredentialing. org/magnet/*.

- Read *From Silence to Voice* (Buresh & Gordon 2006), which is nursing's manual on how to speak out about the life-saving work that nurses do. *From Silence to Voice* provides insight into why nursing has long been invisible to much of the public. It also provides valuable guidance to help nurses get their stories out and increase public respect for their work at this critical time, and gives excellent guidance on how nurses can become more media savvy.

- Become a member of your professional organizations and legislative work groups for healthcare reform to address the image of nursing in the workplace, the public, and the media.

To shape a better image of nursing, take action. Visit the Center for Nursing Advocacy Web site at *www.nursingadvocacy.org* and take a look at the page on taking action. Select some of the ideas presented and help advance a positive, celebratory image of professional nursing. Just a few of the many excellent recommendations are listed here to help you get started:

- Create bulletin boards with nursing research at your workplace.

- Create a dashboard with improved patient care outcomes for specific nurse-sensitive quality indicators and performance measures and display it in high-traffic areas in your practice settings so that everyone—physicians, families, patients, students, and administrators—can see your effect through professional care delivery.

- Post flyers that have positive images of nurses around your workplace and community.

- Do inservices and presentations in your community about the complex roles, levels of expertise, and significant contributions nurses make to healthcare and public safety. Talk about what you do with excitement and energy!

- Invite local high school students interested in healthcare careers to lunch, to educate them about the work of nurses, and to encourage them to experience the full range of nursing opportunities in their own communities.

- Create patient education materials—videos, articles, books, guides, and Web sites. The public needs to know that nurses are health education experts. Write articles for lay magazines, newspapers and books, patient education Web sites, and other publications where patients go to look for health education. Nurses have a unique holistic perspective on healthcare and must establish themselves as reliable patient education professionals.

- Blog about your experiences practicing nursing. Change the image through positive, celebratory examples of how you participated in the healing of others, how you were involved in organizational redesign by participating in a strategic planning session, or how you precepted three brand-new nurses!

- Submit similar stories to your local newspapers so the media can use them to help build their stories from a nursing perspective.

- Start a Nurse Shadowing Program for medical students and interns at your hospital or school. Help educate physicians as to the nature of nursing work, so they can play a more positive role in fostering more collaborative relationships, which lead to better patient outcomes. Dartmouth Medical School and Dartmouth-Hitchcock Medical Center in Lebanon, NH, have started an innovative nurse shadowing program. Read more at *http://dartmed.dartmouth.edu/summer05/html/vs_mantra.php.*

- Create a "Be a Nurse for a Day" program. Ask your local media and potential student nurses to shadow you at work so they can learn what you do and elevate their image of nursing (especially if they already have a positive one). Read more about programs such as this at the Center for Nursing Advocacy's Web site: *www.nursingadvocacy.org/action/follow_a_ nurse.html.*

Strengthen the nursing profession

Here are some more ways you can focus on improving your level of excellence:

- Become certified in your specialty. National certification builds confidence in your professional knowledge, skills, and attitudes, and demonstrates your commitment to excellence in meeting national standards.

- Recruit others into the profession.

- Become a member of your professional organizations, including those in your specialty or subspecialty areas of practice.

- Participate in the MRP journey at your institution.

- Participate in shared governance at your institution.

- Precept and mentor the next generation of nurses.

- Participate in nursing peer review.

Advocate for nursing with your legislators. Learn how with more information at *Advance for Nurse Practitioners;* see *http://nurse-practitioners. advanceweb.com/editorial/content/editorial.aspx? cc = 81728.*

Promote nursing research and evidence-based practice

Excellence in practice requires ongoing focus on staying current with evidence-based nursing practice:

- Attend conferences on nursing research and evidence-based practice.

- Do an online search for nursing research journals to see what types of studies are reported in them. Compare the most current ones with those published 10 and 20 years ago (Flaugher 2008).

- Find out what research is being done in your organization and by whom. Talk with those nurses who are involved, including those on units where research is being done. What do they know about research and evidence-based practice (Beyea & Slattery 2006)? How does their research help nurses become more competent? Or does it?

- Establish and/or participate in a journal club on your unit. Look at articles specific to the patient population you work with every day. What research is being done to improve patient care outcomes as reported in those articles? How can you apply that research to your own practice?

Nightingale was the first nurse researcher. Years ahead of her time in statistical analysis, she compiled data and wrote reports to support each reform she pursued, making her exceedingly successful in her endeavors. This scientific ability, combined with her political connections and influence, led to many additional reforms through the governing subcommissions she helped create, including establishing a Statistical Department of the Army, instituting an Army Medical School, and reconstructing the Army Medical Department (Schuyler 1992).

Florence Nightingale replaced the image of nursing as one practiced by the uneducated and inept—though "kindly and attentive"—caregivers with one that exemplifies the tenets of profession-alism published in the first nursing textbook (1859). The literature is filled with examples and renderings of her far-reaching legacy and an enduring image of professional nursing. The school of nursing she established in 1860 still stands today. Believing that problems associated with poverty could be resolved only when people were educated to govern themselves, she supported bills for increased self-government and improved local education.

Today nurses must also have a powerful voice and recognize that hardwiring excellence into our nursing practice will greatly affect nursing's image. Nursing excellence lies in professional nursing practice made visible to those who serve and to those who serve with them.

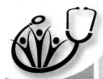

NURSING VOICES

Personal Perspectives: Recently Graduated Nurse

By Tanya Becks, RN

My view of nursing's image—and how it has changed now that I'm in the "real world."

What is it to be a nurse? What exactly is a nurse? What is the image of nursing to me? These are all questions I mull over from time to time, especially when people ask me what my job is, and what exactly I do.

Nurses are people who provide care and comfort to others who need it. We are educated individuals who work together as a team to manage the treatments and care that patients need. Nurses are essentially the glue that holds the healthcare team together.

The image of nursing is important for several reasons. One reason is to hold high the standard of care we provide for our patients and for each other. Another reason is to foster mutual respect with our patients and our fellow healthcare workers.

The image of nursing is shaped by how we nurses portray ourselves as professionals, and it also includes the perceived image held by the general public. My view of the

The Image of Nursing

NURSING VOICES

image of nursing has evolved in the transition from student nurse to graduate nurse and then to registered nurse. As a student, I felt strongly about portraying the nurse's image in a positive light. I entered nursing school very "green" and naïve to all that being a nurse entails. I knew that having a good understanding of science and math coupled with being a caring person would be a good foundation for a nursing career. I also knew that being a nurse meant I would be able to live anywhere in the world and have a job to support myself. As I continued on through nursing school and got involved in community activities on and off campus and in nursing organizations, my pride in being a nurse grew. With this pride came a better understanding of why the image of nursing is so important—both for nurses and for everyone who isn't a nurse, if for nothing else than to be taken seriously as a member of such a noble profession.

Now that I have finished school and am working as a nurse at a local hospital, the image of nursing is more important to me than ever! Being a nurse is hard, and it can be very intimidating. No class at school can truly and fully prepare a nursing student to "be a nurse." Being a nurse is an evolution, a process. It is important to me to portray nursing as a noble profession. We have the privilege of touching people's lives in an intimate way, at their most vulnerable moments. Not only are we touching lives, we are also managing the care and treatments of these people, our patients.

Tanya Becks is a registered nurse currently working and residing in Michigan. As a student nurse at Lansing Community College, she traveled to Africa to perform cardiovascular screenings in a village in Ghana. She is pursuing graduate studies with an emphasis on natural therapies and community health.

REFERENCES

American Nurses Credentialing Center (2005). *The Magnet Nursing Services Recognition Program for Excellence in Nursing Service, Health Care Organization, Instructions and Application Process Manual.* Washington, DC: American Nurses Credentialing Center.

Beyea, S.C., & Slattery, M.J. (2006). *Evidence-Based Practice in Nursing: A Guide to Successful Implementation.* Marblehead, MA: HCPro, Inc.

Buresh, B., & Gordon, S. (2006). *From Silence to Voice: What Nurses Know and Must Communicate to the Public* (2nd ed.). Foreword by Patricia Benner, RN, PhD, FAAN. Ithaca, NY: ILR Press, an Imprint of Cornell University Press.

Chitty, K.K., & Black, B.P. (2007). "Chapter 3: The professionalization of nursing." In *Professional Nursing: Concepts & Challenges* (5th ed.). St. Louis, MO: Saunders Elsevier.

Cohn, K.H. (2007). *Collaborate for Success! Breakthrough Strategies for Engaging Physicians, Nurses, and Hospital Executives.* Chicago, IL: Health Administration Press.

Felgen, J. (2007). I_2E_2: *Leading Lasting Change.* Minneapolis: Creative Health Care Management.

Flaugher, M. (2008). *Nursing Research Program Builder: Strategies to Translate Findings into Practice.* Marblehead, MA: HCPro, Inc.

Gordon, S. (2005). *Nursing Against the Odds: How Health Care Cost Cutting, Media Stereotypes, and Medical Hubris Undermine Nurses and Patient Care.* Ithica, NY: Cornell University Press.

Guanci, G. (2007). *Feel the Pull: Creating a Culture of Nursing Excellence.* Minneapolis: Creative Health Care Management.

Harrington, L.C., & Smith, M. (2008). *Nursing Peer Review: A Practical Approach to Promoting Professional Nursing Accountability.* Marblehead, MA: HCPro, Inc.

Koloroutis, M. (Ed.). (2004). *Relationship-Based Care: A Model for Transforming Practice.* Minneapolis: Creative Health Care Management.

McClure, M., & Hinshaw, A.S. (Eds.). (2002). *Magnet Hospitals Revisited: Attraction and Retention of Professional Nurses.* Washington, DC: American Nurses Publishing.

Nightingale, F. (1859). *Notes on Nursing: What It Is, and What It Is Not.* London: Harrison and Sons, Bookseller to the Queen.

Schuyler, C. (1992). "Florence Nightingale: Commentary on Notes on Nursing." In commentaries section of *Notes on Nursing by Florence Nightingale.* Philadelphia: Lippincott Williams & Wilkins.

Swihart, D. (2006). *Shared Governance: A Practical Approach to Reshaping Professional Nursing Practice.* Marblehead, MA: HCPro, Inc.

Code of Ethics for Nurses: An Image of Professional Integrity

By Diana Swihart, PhD, DMin, MSN, CS, RN-BC

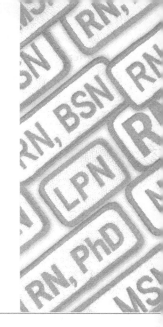

After reading this chapter, the participant will be able to:

✔ Analyze the ethical responsibilities of nursing

✔ Determine how nursing ethics relate to professionalism

✔ List strategies for promoting an ethical image of nursing

Ethical, Professional, and Legal Obligations for Nursing

Nurses today serve on ethics committees, write books and articles about ethics, and obtain advanced degrees in ethics. Why? Because now, perhaps more than at any other time in history, nurses confront a growingly complex array of ethical dilemmas—the "gray areas" between competing right decisions—and the challenges they present, including:

- Human, material, and financial resources

- A global nursing and nurse educator shortage

- Confidentiality and information sharing in an age of technology

- Scientific and technological advances in healthcare options

- Diverse levels of education and skill sets of healthcare providers

- Patient and employee safety (e.g., medical errors, impaired caregivers, expedience)

- Abusive and/or intimidating behavior among healthcare providers

- Ethnic, cultural, and spiritual diversities among patients and staff

- A flawed or incomplete image of professional nursing

Such challenges have brought ethicists, lawyers, legislators, regulating agencies, theologians, and philosophers to the bedside to argue ethics, guidelines, regulations, and collective decision-making around patient rights and autonomy. Though well-intended, all of these voices need to be filtered when applied to practice settings. Nurses filter obstacles, challenges, and competing demands to determine what is right and wrong for their patients and themselves when administering their responsibilities every day.

As scientific and technologic advances become more sophisticated, the ethical decisions they demand become more complex. The field of bioethics has evolved with organized concepts and ways of thinking about ethical dilemmas. The American Nurses Association developed the *Code of Ethics for Nurses* to help them navigate the sometimes murky waters of ethical decision-making that they encounter in the workplace.

State board of nursing practice standards relating to ethics

The state nurse practice act is one of the most important laws in place governing autonomous nursing. Professional nurse practice acts are state regulatory law, statutes passed into law to control or regulate entities or individuals that the government has the right to oversee. State legislatures pass professional practice acts to protect the public, enforce acceptable standards of practice, and authorize boards of nursing to enforce the laws regulating nursing practice (Rothman 2003). Each state professional practice act exercises "police powers," an ability to regulate professional practice that is absolute. Consequently, professional practice acts are inconsistent from state to state and discipline to discipline. For example, enforcement regulations, the powers and roles given to each regulatory agency delegated the responsibility to administer and enforce the act, and the rights and obligations of the licensee can vary significantly.

Currently, though, all states mandate licensure of professional and practical nurses following the successful passage of licensure exams for the registered nurse (RN) and the licensed practical nurse (LPN) or licensed vocational nurse (LVN). Other similarities in practice acts include the "Definitions Section" (or sections) explaining how to interpret the terms used in the text of the act, such as *Board of Nursing*, *physician*, *direct supervision*, *what can and cannot be delegated*, and *approved program of professional nursing education*. This section always includes the definitions of licensed practical or vocational nursing practice, professional nursing practice, and/or advanced practice nursing, unless the state has passed separate practice acts for any of these practice groups. Some state practice acts also define certified nursing assistants (e.g., Florida).

Definitions of practice provide the legal foundation for nursing practice in each state. Many definitions broadly reflect an expanded, ever-changing scope of practice. Others are more restrictive. Therefore, every nurse must adhere to the state's definition of the practice of nursing applicable to his or her academic preparation and experience to be legally safe when providing patient care in his or her state.

Most boards of nursing have been legislated fairly extensive power to enforce nurse practice acts through different types of discipline. The reasons for initiating a disciplinary proceeding are based on a nurse's ability to practice with skill, care, and competence and may include:

- Conviction of a crime, especially if the crime is directly related to the practice of nursing

- The willful failure to report child or elder abuse as required by state law

- The falsification of any document relating to the practice of nursing

- Use of or addiction to alcohol or drugs that affects the nurse's ability to practice safely

- Disciplinary action in another state that is similar or substantially similar to that for which the nurse can be disciplined in the current state of licensure

- A willful or negligent breach of nurse-patient confidentiality

- A willful or negligent breach of ethical conduct, such as:

  - Inappropriate sexual relations with a patient

  - Sexually harassing a patient or a staff member

  - Discriminating against a patient based on ethnic, religious, or other background or characteristics

  - Cheating on a nurse licensing exam

Some nursing boards have even incorporated a code of ethics, such as the American Nurses Association's *Code for Nurses*, into the practice act as part of their rules to enforce the nurse practice act (e.g., Illinois). This emphasizes the importance of ethics in professional nursing practice and demonstrates how the image of nursing is represented in the codes of ethics and conduct.

All ethics and codes of conduct are built on general and fundamental principles that are universal. The major cornerstones of bioethics are respect for autonomy, beneficence, nonmaleficence, and justice, concepts that have always been embedded in nursing. Scientific and technologic advances in healthcare require that nurses expand their instinctive understanding of ethics into one of reasoned and deliberate knowledge that is articulated in evidence-based practice (Jech 2006).

Key Concepts in Ethics

The following is a brief overview of some key ethical concepts: autonomy, justice, fidelity, beneficence, nonmaleficence, veracity, a standard of best interest, obligations, and rights.

- **Autonomy**—the right to self-determination, independence, and freedom, i.e., a nurse's willingness to respect patients' rights to make decisions about and for themselves, even if he or she disagrees with those decisions. This is not an absolute right. Limitations can be imposed when one person's autonomy interferes with another's rights, health, or well- being.

- **Justice**—the obligation to be fair to all people. *Distributive justice* specifically states that people have the right to be treated equally regardless of race, sex, marital status, age, social standing, medical diagnosis, economic level, or religious belief.

- **Fidelity**—the obligation to be faithful to commitments made to self and others. This is the main support for the concept of accountability.

- **Beneficence**—views the primary goal of healthcare as doing good for the patients under one's care. This is more than just technically competent care. Generally, "good" care requires that the healthcare provider approach the patient in a holistic manner, addressing the person's beliefs, wishes, and emotions, as well as those of the families and their significant others.

- **Nonmaleficence**—this is the requirement that healthcare providers do no harm, either intentionally or unintentionally. This may be violated, though, e.g., a patient may undergo a painful and traumatic surgery in order to prolong his or her life. The principle of nonmaleficence also requires that healthcare providers protect those from harm who cannot protect themselves, i.e., mentally incompetent or unconscious patients. Negligence would count as a breach of this principle.

- **Veracity**—"truthfulness" requires that the healthcare provider tell the truth and not intentionally deceive or mislead patients, families, or other healthcare providers. Discomfort or compassion is not a good enough reason to avoid telling patients the truth about their treatment, prognosis, or diagnosis. The patient has the right to factual information that will allow him or her to accurately participate in decision-making about his or her treatments and care.

- **Standard of best interest**—the decision made about a person's healthcare when he or she is unable to make an informed decision for his or her own care. It is based on what the healthcare team and/or family decides is best for that person (e.g., living will). This decision is based on the principle of beneficence. A unilateral decision that disregards the patient's wishes is *paternalism* and may be considered unethical.

- **Obligations**—demands made on persons, professions, society, or government to fulfill and honor the rights of others: (a) *Legal obligations* are formal statements of law and enforceable by law. (b) *Moral obligations* are based on moral or ethical principles and are not enforceable by law.

- **Rights**—are defined as just claims or titles: (a) *Welfare rights* (or *legal rights*) are based on legal entitlement to some good or benefit. (b) *Ethical rights* (or *moral rights*) are based on moral or ethical principles. (c) *Option rights* are based upon a fundamental belief in the dignity and freedom of human beings. These rights allow for freedom of choice.

Laws are the rules of societal conduct based on concerns for fairness and justice that are devised by people to protect society. The goal is to promote peace and productive interactions between people by preventing the actions of one citizen to infringe on the rights of another. *Ethics* declare what is right and wrong—and what ought to be. They are usually presented as systems of valued behaviors and beliefs. Ethics serve to govern conduct to ensure the protection of an individual's rights. Bioethics generally refers to the system of valued behaviors and beliefs held by healthcare workers and organizations.

A *code of ethics* is the written composite of a profession's values and standards of conduct, i.e., the ANA *Code of Ethics*. An *ethical dilemma*, then, is a situation that requires a person to make a choice between two equally unfavorable alternatives. By its very nature, there is no one good solution. The decision made usually has to be defended against those who disagree with it.

ANA's Code of Ethics

A code of ethics has long been the hallmark of professions, including nursing. It is a tool used to define the boundaries and possibilities of practice. It is an implied contract that informs the public and other professions of the rules and principles that govern decisions and by which nurses function (Chitty & Black 2007). The code of ethical conduct:

- Defines professional behaviors and occupational identity

- Promotes safe and competent standards of practice

- Describes the fundamental values and commitments of professionals

- Provides a benchmark for self-evaluation

- Establishes a framework for professional responsibilities and accountabilities

The present-day context of nursing practice places a new emphasis on nursing advocacy and evidence-based care. The American Nurses Association (2001) *Code of Ethics for Nurses with Interpretive Statements* and the *Guide to the Code of Ethics for Nurses: Interpretation and Application* (Fowler 2008) provide nurses with a deeper understanding of the ethical principles that govern the profession. Nurses clarify their thinking and the intent of their decisions around ethical issues and dilemmas when they engage in reflective discussions around them and participate in nursing ethics committees.

The *Code of Ethics for Nurses with Interpretive Statements* (ANA 2001) has nine provisions that describe the fundamental values and commitments of the nurse, the boundaries of duty and loyalty, and nurses' duties beyond individual patient encounters.

Please note: Figure 9.1 is only an introduction to the components of the *Code of Ethics for Nurses with Interpretive Statements* (ANA, 2001). It is strongly recommended that every practicing nurse, student nurse, and faculty member who presumes to teach nurses academically and/or through staff development activities have his or her own copy and reflect on it as often as possible. The image of professional nursing with integrity and ethical purpose is articulated in the tenets of this document and applied to all practice settings.

FIGURE 9.1   KEY TENETS OF THE ANA'S CODE OF ETHICS

Provision	ANA (2001) statement	Emphasis
Provision 1.	The nurse, in all professional relationships, practices with compassion and respect for the inherent dignity, worth, and uniqueness of every individual, unrestricted by considerations of social or economic status, personal attributes, or the nature of health problems.	• Respect for human dignity • Relationships to patients • The nature of health problems • The right to self-determination • Relationships with colleagues and others
Provision 2.	The nurse's primary commitment is to the patient, whether an individual, family, group, or community.	• Primacy of the patient's interests • Conflict of interest for nurses • Collaboration • Professional boundaries
Provision 3.	The nurse promotes, advocates for, and strives to protect the health, safety, and rights of the patient.	• Privacy • Confidentiality • Protection of participants in research • Standards and review mechanisms • Acting on questionable practice • Addressing impaired practice
Provision 4.	The nurse is responsible and accountable for individual nursing practice and determines the appropriate delegation of tasks consistent with the nurse's obligation to provide optimum patient care.	• Acceptance of accountability and responsibility • Accountability for nursing judgment and action • Responsibility for nursing judgment and action • Delegation of nursing activities
Provision 5.	The nurse owes the same duties to self as to others, including the responsibility to preserve integrity and safety, to maintain competence, and to continue personal and professional growth.	• Moral self-respect • Professional growth and maintenance of competence • Wholeness of character • Preservation of integrity
Provision 6.	The nurse participates in establishing, maintaining, and improving healthcare environments and conditions of employment conducive to the provision of quality healthcare and consistent with the values of the profession through individual and collective action.	• Influence of the environment on moral virtues and values • Influence of the environment on ethical obligations • Responsibility for the healthcare environment
Provision 7.	The nurse participates in the advancement of the profession through contributions to practice, education, administration, and knowledge development.	• Advancing the profession through active involvement in nursing and in healthcare policy • Advancing the profession by developing, maintaining, and implementing professional standards in clinical, administrative, and educational practice • Advancing the profession through knowledge development, dissemination, and application to practice
Provision 8.	The nurse collaborates with other health professionals and the public in promoting community, national, and international efforts to meet health needs.	• Health needs and concerns • Responsibilities to the public
Provision 9.	The profession of nursing, as represented by associations and their members, is responsible for articulating nursing values, for maintaining the integrity of the profession and its practice, and for shaping social policy.	• Assertion of values • The profession carries out its collective responsibility through professional associations • Intraprofessional integrity • Social reform

Recognizing specialty ethics

Nursing encompasses autonomous and collaborative care of all individuals in all practice settings and environments of care. Nurses promote health; aid in preventing or mitigating illness and pain; and care for those who are ill, disabled, and dying. They advocate for patients' rights and services, promote a safe environment, engage in nursing and medical research, participate in shaping health policy, manage patient and healthcare systems, and educate interprofessionally (International Council of Nurses 2003). The ANA *Code of Ethics* (2001) applies to direct care nurses and those in advanced practice and nursing specialties with the same moral, ethical, and legal integrity. The primary difference lies in scope of practice and extent of accountability.

Certification, as defined by the American Board of Nursing Specialties (ABNS), is the formal recognition of the specialized knowledge, skills, and experience demonstrated by the achievement of standards identified by a nursing specialty to promote optimal health outcomes. State licensure provides the legal authority for an individual to practice professional nursing. However, private voluntary certification obtained through individual specialty nursing certifying organizations reflect achievement of a standard beyond licensure for specialty nursing practice, carrying with it greater ethical responsibility for practice and outcomes (ABNS 2004) as determined by the guidelines of nursing specialty organizations, the ANA *Code of Ethics*, and state nurse practice acts.

Certification by an accredited agency, such as the American Nurses Credentialing Center or the American Association of Critical-Care Nurses, assures the public that the nurse has maintained a level of knowledge in his or her specialty with ongoing participation in activities that support the maintenance of competence in that specialty. Therefore, the public's image of specialty nurses carries a higher expectation of excellence, professionalism, and ethical conduct than might be expected of other healthcare providers.

The American Nurses Credentialing Center's Magnet Recognition Program®, the gold standard for nursing excellence globally, reflects the true nature of nursing. The image of professional integrity is imprinted upon the student nurse and realized in the graduate. Certification and nursing specialty advance that image to the public, administrators, and other healthcare providers, an image of nurses who are deeply ethical, committed professionals dedicated to the systems and processes improvements needed to deliver optimal patient care across disciplines and practice settings.

Ethics committees

Ethics committees protect patients by helping healthcare providers, patients, and families work through dilemmas so they can make informed choices. They write policies to ensure patients are heard, that they are treated with equity and justice, that their decisions are respected, and that choices made for those with limited or no decision-making capacity reflect their best interests.

Nursing ethics committees, which are usually separate from the hospital's interdisciplinary ethics committee, can help nurses understand the ethical issues that they deal with in their own practice and give them valuable education and support, enhance ethical decision-making, improve reasoning and patient advocacy skills, increase sense of personal satisfaction, learn to analyze cases, interpret and resolve dilemmas, and develop an interdisciplinary voice for addressing ethical issues/concerns.

Both types of ethics committees provide forums

in which to reflect on and reexamine values. Nurses' presence and roles on interprofessional and interdisciplinary ethics committees are vital because they have close, continuous contact with patients. Nurses can advocate intelligently for patients and make a valuable contribution to ethics committees.

The Process of Ethical Decision- Making

Ethical decision-making processes are in place to protect patients' rights of self-determination and their well-being. Three factors guide informed decision: (a) patients must have decision-making capacity, (b) their decision must be voluntary, and (c) they must receive all necessary, relevant information involving the decision and how it will affect them (Jech 2006).

At times, healthcare providers are faced with seemingly unsolvable ethical dilemmas about decisions involving individual patients. Discussion with the institution's ethics committee can help clarify the dilemma and provide options. Some of the ethical issues to consider when resolving these dilemmas can be found in Figure 9.2. Figure 9.3 will guide you through strategies to resolve dilemmas.

FIGURE 9.2   ETHICAL ISSUES TO CONSIDER

Issues of principle	Autonomy; self-determination of patients and professionals; do good; do no harm; justice; fairness; truth-telling; informed consent; quality of life/sanctity of life; the "Golden Rule" of "do unto others as you would have them do unto you"
Issues of rights	Right to privacy; right to decide what happens to one's self/one's body; right to healthcare; right to information; right to choose who you care for; right to live/to die
Issues of duties/obligations	Respect persons; be accountable for decisions/actions; maintain competence; exercise informed judgment in nursing practice; implement and improve standards of nursing; participate in activities contributing to nursing's knowledge base; safeguard clients from incompetent, unethical, or illegal practice of any person; promote efforts to meet public health needs; participate in formulating public policy
Issues of loyalty	Employee-patient relationship; employee-employer relationship; employee-nurse/doctor/other professional relationship; employee–family of patient relationship
Issues of concern in life cycle	Contraception and sterilization; genetic engineering and embryo transfer; abortion; stem cell research; infanticide; adolescent sexuality; allocation of scarce resources; lifestyle; euthanasia

FIGURE 9.3   HANDLING ETHICAL DILEMMAS IN 10 STEPS

1. Review the ethical dilemma to determine all aspects of the issue(s) of concern: health problems, decision needed, ethical components, and key individuals. What are the health problems in the situation? What decision(s) need to be made? What are the ethical and scientific components of the decision? What individuals are involved in or affected by the decision(s)?

2. Gather additional information to clarify all components of the situation. What further information is needed? What can be obtained?

3. Identify the specific ethical issues present. What are the issues of principle, of ethical rights, of ethical duties/obligations, of ethical loyalty, of concern in the life cycle? What are the historical, philosophical, and theological dimensions?

4. Define personal and professional moral positions, both positive and negative. What are your personal values on the issues? What are your professional values? What guidance does the code of ethics for your service offer?

5. Identify moral positions of key individuals, both positive and negative. Why bother with the moral positions of others? How does one identify value positions of others?

6. Identify all value conflicts, if applicable. What are the conflicts within individuals, between individuals, among groups? What about conflicting loyalties? What is the value hierarchy (which value is most important to you right now)?

7. Determine who should make the final decision(s). Who owns the problem? Who decides who decides? What is the role of the healthcare employee?

8. Create an action plan with a range of actions, anticipated outcomes, and responsible agent. What are the alternatives? What are the anticipated outcomes of each possible alternative?

9. Evaluate results of decision/action. Which outcomes will produce the greatest amount of pleasure or good for the greatest number of individuals involved or affected? Which actions conform to ethical principles, which do not, and which are in conflict? To what extent does this action reflect the original intent of nature or the will of God? What are the relative weights of the goods and the harms?

10. Debrief the ethical dilemma and outcomes. Did the decision/action produce the intended results? Is another action needed? What information is transferable to other situations? How can this information be shared with other healthcare providers to help them improve their ethical decision-making skills?

There are no easy answers. Decisions made by and on behalf of patients can profoundly affect their lives and those of their families. Nurses must participate in the process of ethical decision-making to advocate for patients' self-determination and protect their well-being. They assess their patients' decision-making capacity and know generally what to do in borderline cases. They are often cast in the role of the surrogate decision-maker for patients without capacity and need to know how a case referred to the ethics committee is analyzed.

Integrated ethics

Historically, ethical dilemmas have been dealt with on a case-by-case basis, leaving many healthcare providers overwhelmed and confused about what protocols they should follow. The IntegratedEthics program is an innovative national education and organizational change initiative by the Veterans Health Administration (VHA) designed to infuse a clear and consistent process for ethical decision-making and transform traditional ethics committees into integrated programs that better meet the challenges of today's complex healthcare environment. The initiative offers a systematic, comprehensive approach and a wide variety of tools to improve ethics quality in healthcare and more information can be found at *www.ethics.va.gov/ ETHICS/integratedethics/index.asp.*

An integrated ethics program will provide clear structures for dealing with ethical concerns for people in all areas, from patients to practitioners to the most senior leadership. This clear structure is formed by four program elements. The goal of the integrated ethics program is to build on these four elements to continuously improve ethics quality.

- Alignment between standards and practice through an infrastructure that fosters integration between ethics activities throughout the organization;

- A clearly defined approach to ethical cases that arise in the clinical setting;

- A strategy for responding to recurring ethical cases on a systems level; and,

- Ongoing assessment to evaluate ethics quality.

Strategies for Living and Practicing Ethically

Promoting a professional image of nursing means incorporating ethics into everyday practice. Walk the Talk has published some excellent guides for integrating ethics into everyday practices (Harvey & Airitam 2002; Harvey, Smith & Sims 2003). Following are adaptations of some of the many strategies they provide.

Personal commitments

Focus on your ethical image by practicing the following standards:

- Honor your promises and commitments.

- Do business "in the open" unless it involves strategic or confidential information.

- Eliminate offensive words and comments from your vocabulary. They are degrading and unethical and could have legal repercussions.

- Say no to negativity. It is counterproductive, erodes integrity, and sometimes fosters illegal acts.

- Tame the blame. Assigning blame is destructive; switch to problem solving.

- Embrace racial, cultural, and creative diversity.

- Maintain confidentiality.

- Don't confuse cutting corners with efficiency, and strive for efficiency.

- Recognize others' efforts, contributions, and ethical behaviors.

- Practice patience, understanding, and empathy without judging too quickly.

- Talk with people, not at them and never about them.

- Make it safe for others to accept your care and services.

- Focus on serving your patients, their families, and other healthcare team members.

- Obliterate obstacles to ethical practice that you identify or anticipate.

- Make it safe to be ethical.

- Include ethics in performance feedback.

- Celebrate integrity and ethical behaviors.

- Model ethical behavior. Realize how important ethical behavior is and act, regardless of what others choose to do or not do.

(Adapted from Harvey & Airitam, 2002)

Leaders

Leaders can promote an ethical image by concentrating on the following:

- Build values and ethics awareness. Communicate shared values, operating principles, and ethical standards at all levels of the organization.

- Hold people accountable. Demonstrate zero-tolerance for ethics violations.

- Lead by example.

- Use values to drive decisions. Apply unit and organizational values and guiding principles when making decisions. Ethics are displayed in every decision and act.

- Ensure in-sync policies and practices. Make sure rules and standards support the unit and organizational values and ethics.

- Provide values and ethics education to help individuals translate good beliefs into ethical behaviors and responses.

- Pay attention to perceptions, which become reality when it comes to ethics and integrity.

- Focus on steady, incremental change. Ethics and values-alignment are sum total outcomes that rely on lots of improvements in lots of areas.

- Hire and promote ethical people who use the organization's mission, vision, and values as criteria for making decisions; people who believe in ethical principles and act with integrity, who practice uncommon decency in all that they do.

- Encourage initiative. Motivate others to step up and lead ethically rather than waiting for others to do so, complaining, blaming others, or indulging passive-aggressive behaviors.

(Adapted from Harvey, Smith & Sims 2003)

Critical-thinking exercises

Select one of the reflective discussion topics below. Consider the role of nursing in addressing the questions or in thinking beyond those asked. How does your understanding of ethical issues and how you communicate that understanding affect the image of nursing within organizations and communities? Explore the possibilities and discover the extraordinary in the ordinary activities of ethical professional nursing practice.

- **Shared decision-making with patients:** How well does your facility promote collaborative decision-making between clinicians and patients?

- **Decision-making capacity/competency:** Describe what ability patients have to make their own healthcare decisions.

- **Informed consent process:** How does your organization provide information to the patient or surrogate, ensuring that his or her decision is voluntary, and document the decision? How does this differ from informed consent for research?

- **Surrogate decision-making:** Selection, role, and responsibilities of the person authorized to make healthcare decisions for the patient. What role does nursing have in this process?

- **Advance care planning:** What statements made by a patient with decision-making capacity regarding future healthcare decisions might you expect to act on as part of the interdisciplinary care team?

- **Limits to patient choice (e.g., choice of care setting, choice of provider, a demand for unconventional treatment):** How might you respond to these limits and still encourage autonomy in patient care?

- **Ethical practices in end-of-life care:** How well does your facility address ethical aspects of caring for patients near the end of life?

- **Professionalism in patient care:** How well does your facility foster behavior appropriate for healthcare professionals? What happens to those who practice unethical behaviors?

- **Truth-telling:** Do you maintain open and honest communication with patients, including disclosing bad news and reporting adverse events? When would you not do so?

- **Difficult patients:** How do you interact with patients who do not adhere to treatment plans or healthcare recommendations or are disruptive?

- **Cultural, ethnic, and religious sensitivity:** How do you interact with people of different ethnicities, religions, cultures, ages, sexual orientations, genders, etc.? Is that different from how you interact with those of similar ethnicities, religions, cultures, ages, sexual orientations, genders, etc.?

- **Ethical practices in resource allocation:** How well do you manage the resources you are allocated for programs, services, and patients? Are you or those you work with ever wasteful of resources or time? How do you justify those behaviors?

- **Leadership:** Describe the behaviors of leaders who support an ethical environment and culture. Is this important? Why or why not?

- **Ethical practices in the everyday workplace:** How well does your facility support ethical behavior in everyday interactions in the workplace? How do you and your coworkers respond to those behaviors?

- **Ethical climate:** Is there openness to ethics discussions, perceived pressure to engage in unethical conduct, and/or the opportunity to engage in ethical conduct among your peers? How would you describe an ethical climate in your facility?

- **Ethical practices in research:** How well does your facility ensure that its employees follow ethical standards that apply to research and evidence-based practices?

(Reflective discussion questions adapted from the Domains of Ethics in Healthcare and the VHA IntegratedEthics Program retrieved online July 3, 2008, from *www.ethics.va.gov/ETHICS/docs/integratedethics/Domains_of_Ethics_in_Health_Care_20071011.pdf.*)

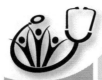

NURSING VOICES

Personal Perspectives: Recently Graduated Nurse

By Tanya Becks, RN

I am very proud to be a nurse, but at the same time I remain humble and realize that I still have so much to learn. I am proud that the career I have chosen is ever-evolving and will require me to stay on my toes, continue to expand my knowledge, and grow personally and professionally as I reach these goals.

I think it is also important to have a sense of humor as a nurse. Rolling with the punches is not always easy, but being able to laugh at ourselves and learn from our mistakes is almost as important as getting through school and passing the board exam. As individual nurses, each of us brings various views, strengths, and gifts to the profession. It pleases me to be a part of a life's work that can use and embrace all of the different gifts we have. The possibilities and opportunities to achieve our goals and dreams are truly endless! Not only am I proud to be a nurse, but I am excited to see where this journey will take me.

REFERENCES

American Nurses Association. (2001). *Code of Ethics for Nurses with Interpretive Statements*. Washington, DC: American Nurses Publishing.

American Nurses Association. (1996). *Model Practice Act*. Washington, DC: American Nurses Publishing.

American Board of Nursing Specialties (ABNS). (2004). "A position statement on the value of specialty nursing certification." Available at *www.nursingcertification.org*.

Beauchamp, T.L., & Childress, J.F. (2001). *Principles of Biomedical Ethics* (5th ed.). New York: Oxford University Press.

Chitty, K.K., & Black, B.P. (2007). *Professional Nursing: Concepts & Challenges* (5th ed.). St. Louis: Saunder/Elsevier.

Fowler, M.D.M. (Ed.). (2008). *Guide to the Code of Ethics for Nurses: Interpretation and Application*. Silver Spring, MD: American Nurses Association.

Harvey, E., & Airitam, S. (2002). *Ethics 4 Everyone: The Handbook for Integrity-Based Business Practices*. Dallas: Walk the Talk Company.

Harvey, E., Smith, A., & Sims, P. (2003). *Leading to Ethics: 10 Leadership Strategies for Building a High-Integrity Organization*. Dallas: Walk the Talk Company.

International Council of Nurses. (2003). "The ICN definition of nursing, 2003." Available at *www.icn.ch/definition.htm*.

Jech, A. O. (2006). "Everyday Ethics for Nurses." Available at *www.nurse.com/ce/60097*.

Montgomery, J.W. (1986). *Human Rights and Human Dignity*. Dallas: Probe Books.

National Center for Ethics in Healthcare. (2007). "IntegratedEthics Initiative." Available at *www.ethics.va.gov/ETHICS/integratedethics/index.asp*.

National Council of State Boards of Nursing (NCSBN). (2004). *Nurse Licensure Compact Rules and Regulations*. Chicago: NCSBN.

Nursing Ethics Network. Availabe at *http://jmrileyrn.tripod.com/nen/nen.html*.

Rothman, D. (2003). *Strangers at the Bedside*. New York: Aldine de Gruytler.

CHAPTER 10

From Voice to Action: How Nurses are Changing Our Image

By Edie Brous, RN, MSN, MPH, JD

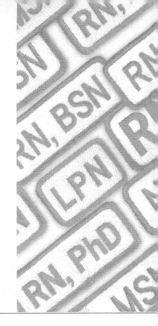

LEARNING OBJECTIVES

After reading this chapter, the participant will be able to:

✔ Explain how media portrayals of nursing influence public opinion

✔ Discuss the role played by the Center for Nursing Advocacy in changing nursing's image

Media Misperceptions

Despite the wealth of research linking nursing to improved patient outcomes, the public remains largely uneducated about the true role nurses play in modern healthcare. Although newspaper articles bemoan the nursing shortage, little is done to explain the reasons behind it or to take responsibility for the media's contribution to it. Attempts to educate the public and the media face an uphill struggle against firmly entrenched hierarchies and marketing practices. The tireless efforts of the Center for Nursing Advocacy reveal what can be done to address this problem.

The pervasive portrayal of nursing in less than accurate lights undermines the profession's ability to convey the reality of the profession to the public. Traditionally, nurses have been cast in inaccurate and unflattering ways. Each of these images conveys the wrong message to the public about nursing's worth. This imagery prevents the profession from being taken seriously as healthcare providers who affect patient outcomes and prevent complications. This imagery also undermines efforts to resolve the global and critical shortage that is currently ravaging public health. And this imagery frustrates attempts to obtain adequate funding for nursing initiatives. As long as nurses are envisioned as baby-hugging pillow-fluffers, the public remains at risk.

Sexualized imagery

Depictions of nurses wearing push-up bras and high heels may satisfy sexual fantasies, but they damage the profession and endanger patients. Bimbos are not taken seriously or funded for their work. The relentless linking of sexual images to nursing conveys the message that nurses serve primarily an erotic purpose. It perpetuates the misconception that all nurses are female, submissive, and sexually available.

In the past few years alone, Dentyne Ice gum, Gillette TAG Body Spray, and Schick Quattro Titanium razors all created advertisements that lured naughty nurses into bed with the men who used their products. Pop star Christina Aguilera played a sadistic naughty nurse in a Skechers print ad for shoes.

Such stereotypical sexualization demoralizes practicing nurses and deters others from considering nursing as a career. A profession that requires education, skill, and expertise appeals to intelligent, ambitious people. When nursing is portrayed in this more professional manner, its ranks will be increased. However, as long as nurses continue to be portrayed as sex objects, intelligent, ambitious people will seek work in other fields.

The perpetual degradation of nursing results in inadequate resource allocation for nursing recruitment, clinical practice, education, and research. In the absence of such resources, dangerous staffing shortages will continue. Such damaging imagery perpetuates the shortage and intensifies the global staffing crisis. The widespread lack of respect for nursing contributes to sexual and physical abuse in the workplace, further eroding the nursing ranks.

Nursing's concern about sexualized imagery stems from a concern for patient welfare, not from a lack of humor or prudishness. The devaluation of nursing has a direct impact on patient welfare because it accelerates the exodus from clinical practice. When patients lose the advocacy of professional nurses, they suffer more complications and die in higher numbers.

Physician extenders

Healthcare-themed television shows do a tremendous disservice to nursing, and by extension, to patients. The viewing public is consistently provided with distorted images of provider roles. All care is physician-centric: Physicians save lives while nurses are blindly obedient and largely peripheral. Physicians are brilliant heroes; nurses are uneducated servants. Physicians have authority over nursing, and are the main and sometimes only providers in hospital settings.

When members of the public are constantly bombarded with these misrepresentations, they develop distorted perceptions of nurses and their contributions. People weighing career options consider nursing to be an unskilled, "girly," low-esteem choice. When nurses are consistently portrayed as mindless handmaidens, the profession loses potential newcomers. If nurses were portrayed as the essential, critical elements in patient safety that they are, the profession would hold more appeal for recruitment.

When television shows depict nurses urgently and blindly following doctor's commands, the public does not see that nurses are independently licensed professionals with a distinct scope of practice. When *ER* depicts nurses only as frustrated physician wannabes or physician helpers, the public does not know that real nurses autonomously perform procedures without physician involvement. Nurses see patients first, triage patients, use their clinical judgment and skills, and perform as a vital team member in saving lives, and they should be portrayed as such.

When *Grey's Anatomy* shows physicians ordering nurses around and physicians acting as nursing administrative supervisors with no nurse managers in sight, the public does not know that nurses are interviewed, supervised, educated, hired, disciplined, and fired by other nurses. The public does not know that nursing is an independent profession completely outside the control of physicians. The media's perpetual depiction of nurses in such a disrespectful manner contributes to the public's anachronistic handmaiden view of nursing. Evidence suggests policymakers share this perception. As long as this is the case, they will continue to drastically underfund nursing and ignore working conditions that endanger both nurses and patients.

Little girls and angels

Although nurses are living, breathing, thinking adults, some coverage of nursing issues and a great deal of marketing tends to be geared toward perpetuating a view of nurses as little girls or angels of mercy. Such angel imagery characterizes nursing work as tender loving care, and nursing roles are reflected as benevolent and emotionally based. These images depict nurses as maternal martyrs, with no human needs and endless capacities for self-sacrifice. While other professionals can expect to be respected and compensated for their abilities, nurses are depicted as noble altruists, dedicating their efforts without concern for their own human needs. Little to no attention is paid to the rigorous academic preparation or licensing requirements to practice nursing.

In 2002, Johnson & Johnson (J&J) launched "The Campaign for Nursing's Future," which had a stated goal of easing the nursing shortage. The campaign's most public efforts have gone into a series of commercials intended to entice people into nursing. The stated goal, however, was undermined by the traditionally sentimentalized, emotional depiction of nurses. Both the 2002 "Dare to Care" and the 2005 "Nurse's Touch" promotions perpetuate the stereotypical imagery of nursing as a field for kind-hearted, compassionate caregivers. These regressive images do not appeal to sophisticated, science-oriented, scholarly, or ambitious people who wish to be taken seriously as professionals.

The advertisements do not focus on nursing skill, knowledge, or judgment, nor do they teach the public about nursing's contribution to patient safety. The campaign relies on traditional "soft" descriptions of nurses "touching lives," when nurses *saving* lives would be more accurate and effective. After the Center and other nursing advocates expressed concerns about the nature of the ads, J&J introduced a new round of commercials in 2007 that commendably highlighted nurses' life-saving value, although they still included some regressive angel imagery that is antithetical to their stated goal.

Although compassion is an essential element in patient care, it is not the *raison d'être* for nursing. Ironically, even manifestations of nurses' life-saving skill may be misconstrued as simple hand-holding. Nurses hold hands to assess body temperature and bilateral limb strength. They bring humor into the workplace to assess level of consciousness and facial symmetry. They talk to patients to assess sensorium and their ability to understand medication and treatment plans. They play with children to assess psychomotor skills, emotional states, and developmental milestones. These activities are not performed out of devotion and affection, but as a required element in patient care. They require more than compassion; they require professional skill and education. These activities that are consistently portrayed as kindness are, in fact, the activities that save lives. They deserve to be respected as such, but instead are characterized as fluffy emotional support. Emotional support is not a virtuous "angel of mercy" activity; it is provided because it improves patient outcomes.

Absence

On April 12, 2007, New Jersey Governor Jon Corzine was in a near-fatal automobile accident. He appeared six weeks later in a public service announcement regarding the use of seatbelts, in which he stated, in part, ". . . I lost over half my blood and broke 15 bones in 18 places. I spent eight days in intensive care where a ventilator was breathing for me. It took a remarkable team of doctors and a series of miracles to save my life . . . "

Governor Corzine (and some news articles covering his crash) did not attribute his survival to the critical care of nurses who monitored that ventilator, along with his breath sounds, level of consciousness, heart tones, bowel and bladder function, fluid and electrolyte balance, acid-base status, etc. The nurses who administered his medications, titrated his intravenous drips, operated the machinery, provided around-the-clock vigilance, etc., were not given any credit. His "remarkable team of doctors" and "series of miracles" did not manage his airway or monitor his urine output and vital signs—the nurses did. His "remarkable team of doctors" and "series of miracles" did not provide 24/7 observation for cardiac arrhythmias, or neurological changes—the nurses did.

This "public service" announcement did not fully serve the public. It conveyed the message that all life-saving is performed by physicians. It ignored the professionals who provided the surveillance that kept Corzine alive, and perpetuated the misconception that nurses are invisible or irrelevant. The physicians were "remarkable," but the nurses were invisible.

The media typically attributes survival or recovery to physicians and miracles, completely ignoring the nurses' contributions to patient outcomes. The absence of nursing in these stories exacerbates the public's inability to recognize nursing's contribution.

Effects of Media Portrayals

As long as the media continues to characterize nursing in such a manner, public policymakers will continue to underfund nursing clinical practice, research, and education. Patients will continue to be the casualties of those funding decisions. As long as the media perpetuates these negative stereotypes, intelligent, ambitious people will veer away from choosing nursing as a career. The shortage will intensify. The public must understand that it is the nurse who stands between them and danger. Movies, television dramas, novels, newspapers, and other media must provide accurate information about nursing instead of perpetuating outdated imagery. It is not simply a morale issue for nurses—it is a grave matter of public health.

The media either distorts, degrades, or ignores nursing. Some make arguments that television shows are fictional, and therefore cannot affect the way people think. But a large body of research shows that fictional shows influence public perceptions of nursing (and other health professionals) and shape health beliefs and behaviors while entertaining viewers. The media's perpetual anachronistic and inaccurate stereotypes damage the profession by creating a false reality. They shape opinions and alter perceptions. Shows like *ER* and *Grey's Anatomy* reach vast audiences across the world and have the ability either to educate or to perpetuate misinformation. Unfortunately, they choose the latter at the expense of patients, who are already suffering the effects of a dangerously shorthanded nursing profession.

Plotlines consistently revolve around physicians, giving the impression that they are the only healthcare providers in a hospital setting. Episodes show physician characters performing work that, in reality, is performed by nurses. Stories do not reflect the critical role nurses play, and thus they present inaccurate portrayals of the healthcare system.

When the viewer is exposed time and time again to images of physicians as brilliant heroes and nurses as mindless servants, sexual bimbos, or tender little girls, the public perception of nursing is damaged, and consequently patients are harmed. Health policy is determined by the public perception of healthcare issues and, as such, it is simply irresponsible to continually depict nursing in such inaccurate and disrespectful fashions.

Nurses need to be a visible presence in the media. The public must know that it is not the physician who is the first responder in an emergency— it is the nurse. The media should educate the public on nursing's real and valuable role in healthcare policy, legislation, research, education, and patient safety instead of continuing its current role of intensifying the undervaluation of nursing.

Young people making initial career choices and mature persons considering second careers will continue to eliminate nursing as an option when the profession is consistently portrayed in an unflattering manner. Pharmaceutical campaigns that urge us to "Ask your doctor" and talk television segments further erode the nursing workforce by relentlessly pushing messages that physicians are the only providers with knowledge and expertise.

The cumulative effect of this relentless antinurse bias undermines nurses currently in practice. Unsafe working conditions are not addressed. Funding remains inadequate. Safe staffing ratios are not assured. Nurses leave the workplace. Experienced providers disappear. The professional skill required for patient safety is eroded. Morbidity and mortality increase. Costly and deadly complications are not prevented.

External Solutions

In 2001, in response to the growing global nursing shortage, a group of seven graduate students at Johns Hopkins University School of Nursing founded the Center for Nursing Advocacy to improve what they perceived to be a lack of public understanding about nursing. The Center soon became a 501(c)3 nonprofit organization working to improve media and other public images of nurses, to foster a dialogue about nursing and its value, and with the overall goal of resolving the global nursing shortage. The Center works to improve the accuracy of information conveyed to the public about nursing, increase the visibility of the nursing profession, and discourage damaging portrayals of nurses. Toward that end, the Center has waged many effective public campaigns. Its hub of action is located online at *www.nursingadvocacy.org*.

The Center performs a valuable media-watch service, evaluating movies, television shows, commercials, books, music, news articles, recruitment materials, and much more. It applauds positive portrayals of the profession and protests damaging depictions. The Center issues Golden Lamp Awards at the end of each year to honor the 10 best and 10 worst media depictions of the year.

In 2004, Skechers shoe company released a print ad featuring pop star Christina Aguilera dressed in a dominatrix nurse outfit. After supporters alerted the Center to this depiction, the Center's director telephoned Skechers to ask that they pull the ad—briefing them fully on how negative images of nursing adversely affect the way society thinks about—and funds—nursing. Skechers refused to pull the ad, so the Center issued an action alert to its news alert subscribers, and over the next two weeks, nursing supporters sent 3,000 e-mails to Skechers. Skechers then relented and pulled the ad.

In 2002, the U.S. Department of Health and Human Services Office of Minority Health (OMH) launched its annual "Take a Loved One to the Doctor Day" campaign to urge ethnic minorities to seek out preventive care on a regular basis. The director of the Center, which was still just forming and composed of a handful of students, telephoned staff at the OMH, but they refused to even consider changing the name of the campaign. As rationale, the OMH staff member cited "focus group testing" that found that the word "doctor" resonated with the public. Yet if the media continues to give the public "doctor, doctor, doctor" all the time, that's what the public will expect. The "Doctor Day" title plainly ignores the contributions of advanced practice registered nurses (APRNs). The title is doubly insulting considering that APRNs are most often the only ones who are willing to treat and provide care to underserved communities that are being targeted by the "Loved One" campaign.

The Center for Nursing Advocacy grew much larger over the following two years, and in response to a request from the American College of Nurse-Midwives (ACNM), the Center launched a letter-writing campaign to the OMH to once again request it change the name of the "Doctor Day" campaign. After over 300 e-mails were sent to OMH by nursing supporters—this time directly to the leaders of the OMH—the director of the OMH agreed to have a telephone call with the Center's director. In the call, he said "Sure, we can change the name of the campaign." Once bureaucratic hurdles were cleared, the OMH changed it exactly to what the ACNM suggested: "Take a Loved One for a Checkup Day," which ignores no healthcare provider. This was a big success for nurses to move even the U.S. government—a body many perceive as so unmovable. And it shows the power nurses have when they work together and speak out.

The Center has also successfully convinced many advertisers to remove or improve products or ads featuring nurses, including Wal-Mart, Disney, Schick, Gillette, Clairol, Cadbury-Schweppes (Dentyne), Heineken, Coors, Tickle, and Constellation Brands, among others. Television shows that feature nurses have incorporated some changes in response to Center letter-writing campaigns, but not enough. Hollywood has been far more reluctant to deviate from their heroic physician narratives, which require that physicians receive credit for the work of all other health professionals.

Many of these successes with the media have been achieved with relatively little effort. A 2006 CVS commercial featuring a pharmacist who twice stated that he had educated a layperson to be a nurse in four hours was pulled with a single (but lengthy) phone call by the Center's director to CVSs

VP of customer service. Other of the above efforts were achieved through similar measures. Nurses can make a difference by speaking out. For so long, nurses have simply accepted the media's image of their profession as something too big to even begin thinking about affecting. Even though it will take a long time, we can do this. As French writer Albert Camus once said of such superhuman tasks, the first thing is not to despair. We can one day achieve a better image of nursing—but to get there, we must all take a personal responsibility to improve nursing's public image and reach out to those who affect it.

The Center has effectively initiated letter-writing campaigns to producers and advertisers responsible for undermining nursing. Commercials and television episodes that sexualize nurses, portray them as handmaidens, misrepresent their true roles, etc., have received scores of protesting letters. In attempting to educate those responsible for such damaging depictions, the Center has been successful in changing or canceling altogether the damaging imagery.

The Center has also attracted global press coverage to its activities, educating the broader public and helping the public reconsider its own assumptions and perceptions about nursing.

Internal Changes

Just as importantly, the Center has educated nurses about the power they wield to hold advertisers, news reporters, and television producers accountable. The Center raises the consciousness of nurses, making them more aware of the pervasive and damaging effects of nursing imagery. Additionally, the Center has attempted to make changes within

nursing. Nurses themselves contribute to the public's inability to value the profession by conveying messages in their dress, manner, and behavior. The Center educates nurses about the impact of unprofessional attire and media invisibility.

Although virginal white pinafores and starched caps may be of a bygone era, a professional appearance should not be. If nurses are to be taken seriously as important providers with critical skills and essential information, they must be distinguished from other healthcare workers. To enjoy the respect to which nurses are entitled, patients must recognize nurses as distinct professionals. Nursing must be proactive in removing the role confusion that patients experience.

Nurses must reach out to work with the media to improve the public's understanding of nursing. Nurses can contact members of their local media to affect how they portray nurses. From health minutes on local radio or television stations, to letters to the editor, op-eds, phone calls to advertisers, books, stories, poems, television scripts, and designing positive Halloween costumes, every nurse or nursing student—or member of the general public—can make a difference.

Yet nurses are extremely reluctant to reach out to the media. Sometimes the Center's director speaks to large groups of people, and she is lucky if even one person signs up to receive the Center's free news alerts. But only nurses can fix our image problem—or the global nursing shortage. The Center has made many changes in the media, sometimes with only a single phone call or e-mail. But we must all confront these challenges as part of our professional responsibility to improve the healthcare our patients receive. Nursing could be so much more effective in reshaping nursing's image if each nurse believed in his or her power to make changes to nursing's image and used that self-confidence to take action.

The Center serves an important role, both externally and from within nursing. Their mission is to advocate for a beleaguered profession and, in doing so, improve patient outcomes. When nurses are empowered, taken seriously as professionals, recognized for their impact on patient safety, and treated with dignity, patients suffer fewer complications. When nursing clinical practice, education, and research are adequately funded, critical staffing shortages will be relieved. When the profession is valued, it will appeal to talented, career-minded men and women. But until the media stops denigrating nurses with its regressive imagery, these goals cannot be achieved. It is not solely a quality of life or morale issue for nurses in the profession; it is a matter of public health and patient safety. With critical, global staffing shortages, it is quite literally a matter of life and death.

CHAPTER 11

Shape Up Your Image: It's Time for an Extreme Makeover

By Shelley Cohen, RN, MS, CEN

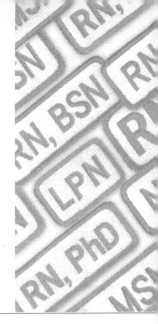

After reading this chapter, the participant will be able to:

✔ Explain ways managers can encourage staff to focus on presenting a positive image

Leaders' and Managers' Role in Promoting a Professional Image

By this time in the text you will have gathered the many perspectives affecting nursing image and the role it plays, both professionally and ethically, in healthcare. Let's take this to the next level, which involves actively engaging in some improvement processes. Is it time for the nursing profession to have its own makeover? Is it time to start saying *no more* to unacceptable representations of the profession? Maybe it is a little of both or a lot of both. It would not hurt for us to give the profession a little tune-up now and then, would it?

But first, let's ask whether we are willing to start with ourselves, to take that individual inventory of how we mirror the nursing profession. Are we willing, as a profession, to truly listen to feedback from our coworkers, patients, and families?

We all try to shape up our physical appearance at one time or another, whether we are male or female. Sometimes we do this with a change in wardrobe or hairstyle. Sometimes we lose weight and focus on a healthier image. Although we're making a change in outer appearance, a new outfit or a slimmer waistline also boosts self-esteem and gives us an air of confidence.

On other occasions, we may make an internal change in our personal attitude that eventually reflects on the outside with a positive change in body language or tone of voice. Maybe we take a course on communication and realize we do not engage in active listening and resolve to change our communication style. The change feels good for us and it feels good for those on the receiving end. As you can see, all of these examples involve the image we present from the inside out.

Action and lack of action, appearance, voice inflection, and an ability to convey empathy and concern all play a role in our image. Where do we begin this makeover process? We begin with one thing and move forward from there, but we do it with intent and a serious attitude.

Four Categories We Can Work On

Let's divide our image makeover into four categories:

1. Professional work environment and interactions

2. Appearance

3. Collegiality/team member role

4. Professional accountabilities

I selected these categories based on the more than 1,000 responses to the survey, along with my personal observations. In further describing examples for each group, I again considered specifics in the survey feedback. Nurses in various areas of the profession—nursing departments, nursing individuals at all levels and practice, nurse faculty, and nursing students—can select a category and develop a program that reshapes their image at the individual or group level.

Professional work environment and interactions

Chapter 6 offered strategies for effective communication, and you can use those strategies both for your personal communication and to set the standard and expectations on your unit. Managers play a key role in creating an environment—you can set expectations for how nurses on your unit will act, communicate, and what achievements and goals are valued.

Use the following tips as criteria for yourself and your staff:

- Do not carry on a discussion in the nurses' station that you would not want others to hear

- Respect the equipment you work with and handle it as if you paid for it out of your paycheck

- Acknowledge people who approach you before they have to ask for your attention

- Support other nurses who are being approached unprofessionally

- Display and advertise your clinical accomplishments

- Follow organizational policy regarding Internet and cell phone usage

- Do not display any behaviors or gestures in view of coworkers, patients, or families that you would not want anyone to see/hear (examples include talking on a cell phone while charting, having an argument with a colleague, or participating in a whining session about the schedule)

Appearance

A good deal of this book has discussed personal appearance, and it's difficult to underestimate its importance to the type of image we portray. Yes, the clothes you choose to wear do not have any bearing on your intelligence, skill as a nurse, or ability to care for your patients. But they do have a bearing on the way you are perceived, and if you do not present an image of professionalism, order, and expertise, your patients will not see past that or recognize that a skilled professional is underneath.

Managers should set expectations for appearance and should never forget to set a good example. Share the following points with your staff:

- Dress for the respect you feel you deserve

- Follow your organizational dress code policies and procedures

- Recognize that your appearance affects perceptions of your competency

- Differentiate yourself in dress from the unlicensed members of your healthcare team

- When not on duty, consider how your appearance still has an effect (e.g., wearing shirts with slogans that imply anything less than professionalism in nursing)

Collegiality/team member role

Everyone knows nursing is a demanding profession, and it belittles our image when we make our job harder by engaging in gossip, backstabbing, or "eating our young." The stresses of the profession are minimized when nurses are able to care for patients in a collegial, supportive environment, where everyone is striving to provide the highest-quality patient care and deliver the best possible patient outcomes.

Set expectations for teamwork and a collegial atmosphere, and keep the following in mind:

- Proactively offer to assist other members of the team to demonstrate team commitment

- Actively become involved in the orientation process of all new staff

- Welcome and accept new staff by communicating your willingness to help them succeed

- Don't allow someone else's unacceptable behavior to become your behavior

- Do not verbally berate another person in your organization

- Be open to constructive criticism and feedback

- Treat all nursing staff—and everyone else who works in the organization—with respect

- Avoid the use of profanity and unprofessional language or gestures

- Support, instead of belittling or chastising, nurses who are expanding their knowledge base with continuing education and/or returning to college

Professional accountabilities

Chapter 8 discussed nursing excellence and the many ways nurses can elevate their practice, through evidence-based practice and nursing research, to joining professional organizations. Be proud of your profession. Hold yourself accountable to high standards.

Managers should set high expectations and share the following with staff:

- Acknowledge that it is your name on your license, not your manager's or your organization's

- Maintain a current knowledge of your nurse practice act

- Belong to and support at least one professional nursing organization

- Maintain a current knowledge base of your specialty through continuing education

- Document appropriately and according to nursing standards of practice

- Adhere to organizational and other practice standards

- Introduce yourself with your name and title (e.g., "My name is Shelley Cohen, and I am your nurse")

TIPS FOR MANAGERS

By Karen L. Tomajan, MS, RN, BC, CNAA, CRRN

The role of the manager is key in promoting a positive image of nursing, both within the organization and in the community. Fostering a positive self-image among the staff is an important first step. Take a look at the tips below.

Promote positive interaction at all levels of the organization

- Promote positive nurse-to-nurse collaboration, and help staff to address conflicts effectively. Address nurse-to-nurse hostility or other instances of unprofessional behavior directly.

- Insist on positive interdisciplinary team interactions.

- Facilitate positive physician relationships. Intervene when negative encounters occur.

- Take every opportunity to model appropriate interactions, with extra attention to difficult individuals or groups.

- Promote assertive communication skills.

- Adopt unit standards for zero tolerance for abuse and consistently enforce these standards.

Promote professional appearance

- Encourage staff to dress professionally.

TIPS FOR MANAGERS (CONT.)

- Consider a standard scrub color for the nurses on the unit. This could help to form a stronger unit identity as well as help identify the nurse to patients, families, physicians, and interdisciplinary team members

- Hold staff accountable for clean, pressed, tasteful uniforms, regardless of the color.

- Require visible identification of the RN or LPN title—on the ID badge, a patch, or other method.

- Promote involvement of staff in determining dress code, as well as active enforcement of established standards.

Promote professional practice

- Help staff take credit for their contributions to positive patient outcomes. Help them articulate the autonomous aspects of their role to patients, families, and the public.

- Set high standards, and serve as a role model in meeting them.

- Help staff members link their personal goals to those of the organization.

- Encourage and support professional development activities: national certification, continued academic education, involvement in professional associations, etc.

- Promote the development of staff expertise in their clinical area. Promote evidence-based practice.

- Recognize the accomplishments of the staff. For example, write congratulatory notes. Alert your supervisor when staff members achieve important milestones so they can also recognize the accomplishment.

Promote a positive workplace

- Provide the tools for staff members to do their job. Ensure adequate staffing, and help staff problem-solve when staffing is not "ideal."

- Use positive language when communicating policy changes or discussing controversial issues. Support your colleague's decisions.

- Monitor staff morale, and work to involve staff in unit decision-making. Carry staff input into organizational decision-making as well.

- Encourage staff participation in organizational initiatives, including employee satisfaction surveys, town hall meetings, quality improvement teams, and committee work.

TIPS FOR MANAGERS (CONT.)

- Promote positive working relationships with nursing schools and students. Monitor student clinical experiences, and intervene if morale issues spill over to the students.By Karen L. Tomajan, MS, RN, BC, CNAA, CRRN

Nurses build the public image of nursing through day-to-day interactions with patients, families, and colleagues. Share the following tips with your staff members on ways they can display a positive image.

Present a professional image

- Make sure your uniform is clean, pressed, and professional. Think about the patterns on your scrub tops—what do they communicate about you?

- Identify yourself as a professional nurse. Keep your name tag visible. Introduce yourself by your full name, and tell patients you are an RN or LPN

- Speak with confidence and self-assurance.

Communicate about your work, and discuss your accomplishments

- Prepare and practice a 30-second "elevator" speech about your role as a professional nurse. Communicate how you have made a difference for patients in your care.

- Describe your independent actions to prevent complications and save lives. Many patients and families believe that all nurses do is follow doctors' orders. When you intervene to address a problem, let them know how your actions made the difference.

- Volunteer to speak about nursing issues, healthcare, or nursing career opportunities to schools or civic groups.

- Provide a great experience for nursing students. Talk to them about your role and your accomplishments as a nurse.

Correct inaccurate nursing stereotypes

- When you see nurses or nursing misrepresented in the media, write a letter to the sponsor or editor.

- You can also work with the Center for Nursing Advocacy to bring even greater attention to the issue.

TIPS FOR MANAGERS (CONT.)

Be engaged in your workplace

- Take opportunities to participate in your employer's opinion surveys. When submitting written comments, take care to provide suggestions for improvement.

- Participate in employee forums, town hall meetings, committees, and other opportunities to become more involved in your organization. Actively engaged nurses experience higher levels of job satisfaction, which improves their sense of well-being.

Grow professionally

- Consider joining and being active in a professional association, whether it is your specialty association, state nurses association, honor society, or all three! Networking and educational opportunities are just the beginning of the benefits of membership.

- Develop a five-year plan for your career. Identify professional development activities that will help you learn the skills necessary to achieve your plan. Seek the input of your manager and the education department of your facility for assistance.

- Watch the legislative agenda at the state and national level. Make calls to your representatives to let them know your opinions regarding healthcare or other issues important to you. Your state nurses association is a good resource for information on legislative affairs.

- Promote positive working relationships within your team. Avoid gossip. If you are having difficulty working with a colleague, approach that individual with your concerns, and work to resolve them. Ask your manager to assist you if you need help preparing for this discussion. You will find that resolving issues proactively helps prevent conflicts from escalating.

If you want to be respected as a professional, it is important that you project your best professional image in every interaction. Respect cannot be demanded; it must be earned. Our image as professionals requires consistent performance every day, by every nurse.

It is an exciting time to be a nurse. Healthcare is changing, and the role and practice of the professional nurse is changing along with it. The value of nurses has been proven and documented. Healthcare organizations are interested in working with their best and brightest nurses to create healthy work environments that will ensure their valued nurses stay with them. Leaders are recognizing that an empowered work force enhances the practice environment and ensures patient safety and positive outcomes.

Take Charge of Our Image

Harvard Business School professor Laura Morgan Roberts tells us, "If you aren't managing your own professional image, someone else is" (Roberts 2005). She also reminds us that we are constantly under observation, which in turn creates perceptions about our competence as well as our character. Begin the process of reshaping our image by selecting one of the categories discussed earlier and initiating improvements. Evaluate how your changes effect what the public sees, hears, and believes about nursing.

Some might say that nursing's problem is a generational issue. Others say that there has been a change in the work ethic across all professions. I have oriented and worked with many new graduate nurses who are 30 years younger than me, some with a great work ethic and some with no work ethic at all. I have worked alongside nurses with the same number of years of experience, and although more of them may have an acceptable work ethic, in no way does this imply that they are nice to be around. Working hard does not make you a good nurse or a good team player. We need to stop accepting one attribute as a minimal expectation of nurses.

Call for Action

Now is the time for a call to action for all nurses, all specialties, all levels of experience and education. For once, we need to agree on what is acceptable for the image of the nurse. To get started as an individual nurse, follow these steps;

- Decide what is acceptable behavior from yourself as a professional

- When you are on and off duty, be proud of what you say, do, and elect not to do

- Introduce yourself as a nurse

- Do a mirror image check before you walk out the door: Are you proud of what you see, or are you just comfortable?

- Brag and brag some more about your accomplishments as a nurse

- Recognize the value you bring to the healthcare system

- Validate your work and value through the documentation process

- Work on your communication style, and ask for feedback to ensure you are leaving a positive reflection

As a professional group we can do even more by:

- Providing scripted responses for nurses to use in response to unacceptable behaviors and verbal intimidations

- Role-modeling the characteristics of a professional nurse

- Requiring our nurse leaders to hold unprofessional nurses accountable

- Working with and supporting our national and local professional organizations

- Going into community groups to clarify and educate the public about the role of the nurse

- Contributing to local and national journalism to ensure that more of the great nurse stories are being told

We could easily fill this book with powerful stories of many grand and some not so grand displays of pride and professionalism. The problem is that people believe what they see and hear, and they need to see and hear more of the greatness of nursing. Starting with any of these categories and beginning the process of reshaping our image will affect what the public sees, hears, and believes about nursing as a profession.

REFERENCES

Roberts, L.M. (2005). "Creating a positive professional image." Available at *http://hbswk.hbs.edu/item/4860.html.*

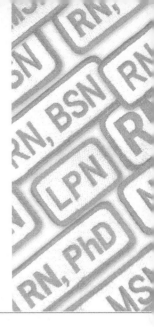

CHAPTER 12

Great Images from Great Nurses

By Shelley Cohen, RN, MS, CEN

LEARNING OBJECTIVES

After reading this chapter, the participant will be able to:

✔ Identify positive examples of nurses in the public eye

✔ Identify ways nursing faculty can shape students' image of nursing

Making a Difference

We are fortunate to have great nurses working in diverse areas of healthcare delivery. You can see these nurses in the office and clinic settings, schools, long-term care areas, home health, prison systems, acute care, pre-hospital care, behavioral health programs, the military, research laboratories, and schools of nursing. Some nurses stand out in the profession because of their role, the publications they have written, a stance they have taken on a public issue, or for a variety of other reasons. What makes these nurses great? Their attitudes, behaviors, and passion for the profession. They recognize that not every day or every shift is going to be easy, but they show up committed to doing what I call the most important characteristic: doing "whatever it takes." They possess a willingness to work alongside peers and other members of the healthcare team to bring effective and quality care to their patient population. They pursue knowledge, role-model professional behaviors, and nourish and support new nurses. These are the characteristics of great nurses.

This chapter focuses on a few of the shining examples of great nurses, including a thoughtful personal perspective from an experienced nursing faculty member on what nursing students think about the profession's image and the role faculty can play in shaping the image of tomorrow's nurses.

Great nurses in history and our own backyard

You can find examples of great nurses throughout history including the courageous Army and Navy nurses stationed in the Philippines in 1941 who ended up in internment camps for several years. These nurses showed great loyalty to their patients while facing starvation and great fear (Norman 1999). The book *We Band of Angels: The Untold Story of American Nurses Trapped on Bataan by the Japanese* shows the inherent ethics that nurses hold as a profession.

Today, as you read this, we have nurses serving the service men and women fighting for our freedoms overseas, and caring for the soldiers back home fighting for their recovery. Each of those nurses brings greatness to those for whom they care. And we have nurses representing our country in our legislative body: we are fortunate to have three nurses serving in the United States Congress. In addition, the acting chief of staff for the Office of the Surgeon General is Rear Admiral Carol Ramon, Chief Nurse for the U.S. Public Health Services.

Closer to home, we all work alongside great nurses in our day-to-day lives. Many states annually nominate great nurses and have ceremonies celebrating their accomplishments. Criteria vary, but always include a common theme of caring and compassion. In northeastern Florida, the campaign for 100 great nurses focuses on those who provide significant care contributions to patients or to the nursing profession. North Carolina's program is directed at those who affect the image and profession of nursing.

Behind the Scenes Greatness

Greatness amongst nurses is not new by any means. The greatness is not just about saving a life in dra-matic scenarios as is too often the sole focus of healthcare on television. For our magnitude is bigger than anything the media can portray. The enormity of what nurses contribute to patients, family, and coworkers is in the behind the scenes actions. Consider these everyday examples of great nurses:

- An emergency room nurse calls her spouse to have him gather up some children's clothes and toys from home and bring them to the ED. The nurse is caring for three siblings recently removed from a meth house who have nothing safe to wear or anything to play with, and the nurse knows it will be hours before Children's Services can sort through placement issues.

- A med-surg nurse knows his out-of-state patient—who is hospitalized with an unexpected medical event—is missing his family. So brings to work an Internet printout of the patient's local newspaper.

- A nurse manager who is working hard to support her staff and develop initiatives that engage nurse empowerment. She tells a physician who displays threatening behavior that he can no longer disrupt her staff with his unacceptable behaviors. The next day the physician sends the manager flowers and thanked her for having the courage to confront him, which he admits should have been done long ago.

- A nurse is confronted with her addiction issues and completes a recovery program. In her third year of recovery, she has made such progress she begins mentoring other nurses experiencing dependence issues.

- A nurse has a family member who is dying of cancer. His coworker volunteers to work an upcoming holiday for him without being asked. The manager swaps the shift so the nurse is surprised the day before the holiday.

- A nurse questions an order by a resident because he had recently read in a nursing journal that the order is contraindicated for his patient. The resident tells the nurse to follow orders, so the nurse pages the attending to discuss his concerns, and the attending changes the order. The patient lives another day.

And then there are the thousands of unnoticed acts that happen every day that are never seen or acknowledged by anyone—not even the nurse who brushes it off as 'part of my job.' These include:

- A nurse who notices a ETOH withdrawal patient does not have an IV, just minutes before the patient's tremors get much worse

- A nurse who catches a medication error made by the physician prescribing morphine for a patient who is extremely allergic to morphine

- A nurse who calls pharmacy to report that the wrong medication has been placed in a medication drawer

Whether it is questioning a medication order, recognizing a clinical red flag alert in a patient, respecting patient privacy, or protecting victims of violence, nurses are at the forefront of immense activities that center around the best interest of patients. Patients are admitted to hospital for nursing care, they go to nursing homes for nursing care, and they call healthcare help lines across the country to receive nursing care. Whether it is delivered in person or using modern technology like telemedicine, the public continues to depend on nursing care.

The American Nurses Association published interpretive statements for its Code of Ethics, which clearly define the ethical standard for nursing. It describes the Code of Ethics as a promise and, as long as the profession exists, the patients we serve depend upon the greatness that comes from the overwhelming responsibilities related to the role of nurses. These include maintaining a current knowledge of diseases, treatments, medications, interventions, and methods of delivering nursing care. This accountability and duty is so great that all states have statutes to direct the care we deliver.

Behind the scenes, every day, each shift, acts of greatness occur among us as nurses advocate for their patients, attend to their emotional and psychological needs, prevent serious errors, and exhibit the high-level critical-thinking skills inherent in the profession.

The greatness of character demonstrated by nurses, the ethical responsibility, and commitment to patient care and safety; these are the images that must be verbalized to the general public if we are to garner the support necessary to preserve and protect this incredible profession. Nursing needs to pledge to continue the greatness of the profession. We do this through the choices we make: our image, our choice.

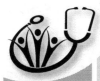

Personal Perspectives: How Students Are Portraying the Image of Nursing

By Richard Freedberg, RN, MSN, MPA

Nurses are seen by the public as honest and trusted professional care providers. That image endures, but it is being shaded and nuanced by the culturally mediated attitudinal shifts that influence those applying to nursing programs. The first item that clearly needs to be articulated is that today's students are, in one sense, a breath of fresh air for nursing's image. Nurses from prior eras were carefully instructed to cultivate a professional distance and avoid self-disclosure of any kind. The lives of my students today are more comfortably integrated into the genuine, multidimensional "self" they bring to class and clinical interactions, with less compartmentalization into "professional," "private," and "social" personae. What you see is what you get. Brightly colored scrubs, athletic shoes, and more engagingly tolerant attitudes have supplanted starched white dress uniforms, the leather shoes, and intransigent, dictatorial care delivery.

The image of nursing my students create also mirrors a change in classroom demographics, which has moved from uniform groups of young white females to cohorts including larger numbers of males, persons from all ethnic minorities, and international students. In addition, I frequently encounter students in their 40s and 50s who've earned prior academic degrees or labored in other careers and have now opted to begin a second, or even third, career as a nurse. Former construction workers, military personnel, lawyers, teachers, microbiologists, social workers, business office managers, and auto plant line workers all have appeared in my class. They bring a broad richness of life experience and diverse worldview to the classroom and hospital.

Present students also bring less desirable characteristics that potentially can bring unfavorable nuances to the public image of nursing. A growing existential pragmatism is one of them. My students lead full and hectic lives. Many are not at all concerned with nursing professionalism and are uninterested in nursing theory. Their ever-present foci are, "What do I need to know for the exam?," "What new skill am I going to learn?," and "How quickly can I get through the program?" There is a predominant egocentrism there that diminishes empathic responses to patients and inhibits acceptance of traditional viewpoints and standards.

As we've seen, current students and recent graduates also look different. The lack of borders between a personal and professional self suggests that new nurses don't necessarily see the value of professional appearance and attire. A random tour of most hospital units will reveal some nurses dressed in rumpled scrubs or a sweatshirt and adorned with visible tattoos and facial piercings. The lack of the customary professional mien is off-putting to a number of patients and can inhibit multidisciplinary interactions with other providers, such as physicians or therapists.

As an additional consideration, the nature of nursing is changing. To be sure, particular elements are timeless, including a professional focus on caring, the therapeutic use of self in client/nurse interactions, and helping people adapt to and cope with the effects of disease. Our clinical role, however, is growing in technical complexity. Also, with the exception of particular subspecialties, such as hospice nursing or extended care settings, our relationships with patients are briefer and often more superficial. This changing face of the practice of nursing offers challenges to preserve the traditional and valued nurse-patient relationship. Applicants transitioning from first or second careers to nursing bring a new perspective. Many of them do not feel a sense of professional duty or mission of caring for those in need. Instead, their compelling interest is stable, predictable employment.

What Can Nursing Faculty Do to Shape the Image of Nursing?

First, we faculty members—particularly those of us who have been nurses for decades—need to not only accept but also embrace cultural change, with all of its wonderful benefits and uncomfortable challenges. We need to work vigorously to ensure that the demographic distribution of our profession mirrors the population from which it is taken. We must actively recruit men, persons of color, and second-career people as students, but also, and perhaps more importantly, as faculty. We can no longer claim to value diversity until our faculty reflects our words.

Culturally diverse and competent nursing faculties then need to continue to create environments in which students can effectively learn to become professional nurses. The current strength of most programs in today's complex healthcare milieu lies in teaching disease process, treatments, procedures, tasks, and the critical-thinking pathway that links this knowledge and guides intervention choices. We churn out technically skilled nurses with a measure of critical-thinking ability. We are perhaps less successful in other dimensions, such as teaching self-awareness and professionalism, and fostering the ability to effectively help design and efficiently deliver interdisciplinary interventions.

Second, nursing faculty must attempt to consciously clarify what "professionalism" denotes and connotes, and assess the relevancy of those meanings and implications within the wider cultural context. We should be asking ourselves which aspects of the

NURSING VOICES

nursing tradition are important and have meaning and what can be left behind. We should identify key attitudes, values, and behaviors, and then determinedly embed them as threads throughout our curricula. It is futile and foolish to focus on superficial accoutrements like clothing and personal adornments without an incessant and aggressive emphasis on helping students gain self-awareness and a firm understanding of how one's personal values and biases direct or shade every interaction with all professional peers and patients.

Third, nursing faculty need to help students acquire empathy and effective communication skills. Regardless of our basic inclination, we faculty ought to accept that both of these characteristics are not innate; they are learned behaviors and can be taught. Each discussion and clinical experience in every course, from nursing fundamentals to critical care nursing, ought to consider self-awareness (what a student brings to the interaction), empathy (an attempt to understand the experience from the patient perspective), and therapeutic communication (the student and patient attempt to come to a shared understanding and goal). If technical expertise and "physical illness" clinical knowledge are two legs of a stool representing nursing professionalism, then self-awareness, empathy, and communication combine to form the third leg.

In summary, nursing can retain and enhance its positive image only if students and faculty conscientiously attend to some basic considerations. Nurses certainly need a comprehensive understanding of disease, treatments, and how patients adapt to both. Nursing schools need to ensure faculty and student populations mirror the larger community, in order to obtain congruency with avowed values. Finally, faculty must recognize that nursing professionalism and patient satisfaction will be achieved only if our students gain self-awareness, empathy, and therapeutic communication skills, in addition to "physical illness" knowledge and skills.

Richard Freedberg has earned an associate's degree in nursing from Lansing Community College, a bachelor of science degree in zoology from Michigan State University, a bachelor of science degree in nursing from University of Detroit–Mercy, a master of science in nursing from Eastern Michigan University, a master of public administration from Western Michigan University, and is a doctoral student in interdisciplinary health studies at Western Michigan University.

His clinical experience includes staff nursing and management roles in medical-surgical and mental health acute care settings, home care nursing, and medical intermediate care. He is currently professor of mental health nursing at Lansing Community College in Lansing, MI. In addition, he continues to practice in a clinical setting.

REFERENCES

American Nurses Association (2001). Code of ethics for nurses with interpretive statements. Silver Spring: Nursesbooks.org.

Norman, E. (1999). *We Band of Angels: The Untold Story of American Nurses Trapped on Bataan by the Japanese.* New York: Pocket Books.

Empowerment Glossary for Nurses

Common words/phrases used by nurses	Replacement power words/statements
Paranoid	Hyper-vigilant
Everyone around here blames everyone else except themselves	Culture of blame
Good patient care	Reaching for nursing excellence
Picked on for doing what is best for my patients	Ridiculed for practicing nursing standards of care
That's the way _____ has always been	I going to speak with _____ about this
I'm just going to check on my patient	I'll be in room _____ if you need me checking BP, neuro status, etc.
Controlling	Authoritative style of leadership
I can't get a break/meal	I'm going to ask the charge to cover for me so that I can take my break
Nothing ever changes around here	I've noticed this subject comes up frequently
It's no use	Let's form a task group to resolve it
I'm sorry to bother you doctor	Dr. Jones, this is Nurse _____ calling to alert you to a clinical change in status for Patient _____ in room 485 . . .
This is how we have always done it	This is an opportunity for improvement
No one notices my contributions	I'd like to share with you how I've handled this situation
I follow doctors orders	I am the first line of defense for the patient and prevent complications and save lives
I am part of a team	I perform independent interventions to protect my patients
It's no use	This is a challenge!
Blame	Accountability
Territoriality	Collaboration
I told them you didn't agree with the new policy, but **they** adopted it anyway	The group discussed your input, and we all decided in the interest of the entire staff and patient care to do _____

Continuing Education
Instructional Guide

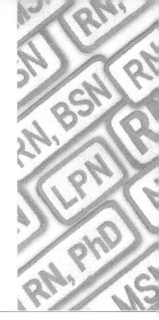

✔ Nurse Managers

✔ Chief Nursing Officers

✔ Chief Nurse Executive

✔ Directors of Nursing

✔ VPs of Nursing

✔ VPs of Patient Care Services

✔ Staff Development Specialists

✔ Directors of Education

✔ Staff Educators

✔ Staff Nurses

Statement of Need

This book and handbook set examines the image of nursing as it stands today and how managers and leaders can improve that image and raise their nursing staff's focus on professionalism. The book discusses how ethics and image are intertwined, and how to shape the image of nursing by focusing on professionalism, autonomy, excellence in practice, and so on. (This activity is intended for individual use only.)

Educational Objectives

Upon completion of this activity, participants should be able to:

- Discuss the current image of the nursing profession

- Recognize the effect of image on public perception

- Discuss the results of a national nursing survey regarding image

- Discuss why the public image of nursing is important

- Explain the reasons why the public image of nursing is different than the reality

- Identify efforts to promote a more accurate public image of nursing

- Discuss the connection between power and image

- Explain how nursing autonomy contributes to professionalism

- Identify why people resist culture change

- Evaluate ways to secure buy-in for culture change

- List reasons why nurses avoid communicating

- Explain how to use the DESC communication model

- Identify characteristics of professional communication

- Identify the Force of Magnetism related to nursing image

- Discuss the role of nursing image in the ANCC Magnet Recognition Program®

- Recognize strategies used by designated organizations to promote nursing staff

- List criteria for judging nursing excellence

- Discuss ways managers can encourage staff to strive for professional excellence

- Analyze the ethical responsibilities of nursing

- Determine how nursing ethics relate to professionalism

- List strategies for promoting an ethical image of nursing

- Explain how media portrayals of nursing influence public opinion

- Discuss the role played by the Center for Nursing Advocacy in changing nursing's image

- Explain ways managers can encourage staff to focus on presenting a positive image

- Identify positive examples of nurses in the public eye

- Identify ways nursing faculty can shape students' image of nursing

Faculty

Shelley Cohen, RN, MS, CEN, is the founder and president of Health Resources Unlimited, a Tennessee-based healthcare education and consulting company (*www.hru.net*).

Kathleen Bartholomew, RN, MN, a registered nurse and counselor, uses the power of story from her experience as the manager of a large surgical unit to shed light on the challenges and issues facing nurses today.

Diana Swihart, PhD, DMin, MSN, CS, RN-BC, is a clinical nurse specialist in nursing education at the Bay Pines VA Healthcare System in Bay Pines, FL.

Laura Cook Harrington, RN, MHA, CPHQ, CHCQM, is the director of live events and continuing education and senior consultant at The Greeley Company, a division of HCPro, Inc.

Barbara J. Hannon, RN, MSN, CPHQ, has been the ANCC Magnet Recognition Program® (MRP) coordinator for the University of Iowa Hospitals & Clinic since 2002.

Karen L. Tomajan, MS, RN, BC, CNAA, CRRN, is the director of nursing quality/special projects at Integris Baptist Medical Center in Oklahoma City.

Edie Brous, RN, MSN, MPH, JD, is a nurse attorney and a board member of the Center for Nursing Advocacy.

Nursing Contact Hours

HCPro is accredited as a provider of continuing nursing education by the American Nurses Credentialing Center Commission on Accreditation.

This educational activity for 3 nursing contact hours is provided by HCPro, Inc.

Disclosure Statements

Shelley Cohen, Kathleen Bartholomew, Diana Swihart, Barbara Hannon, Laura Cook Harrington, Karen Tomajan, and Edie Brous have declared they have no relevant financial relationships to disclose related to the content of this activity.

Instructions

In order to be eligible to receive your nursing contact hours for this activity, you are required to do the following:

1. Read the book

2. Complete the exam

3. Complete the evaluation

4. Provide your contact information on the exam and evaluation

5. Submit exam and evaluation to HCPro, Inc.

Please provide all of the information requested above and mail or fax your completed exam, program evaluation, and contact information to

Continuing Education Manager
HCPro, Inc.
75 Sylvan Street, Suite A-101
Danvers, MA 01923
Fax: 781/639-2982

NOTE: This book and associated exam are intended for individual use only. If you would like to provide this continuing education exam to other members of your nursing staff, please contact our customer service department at 877/727-1728 to place your order. The exam fee schedule is as follows:

Exam quantity	Fee
1	$0
2–25	$15 per person
26–50	$12 per person
51–100	$8 per person
101+	$5 per person

CONTINUING EDUCATION EXAM

Name: _____

Title: _____

Facility name: _____

Address: _____

Address: _____

City: _____ State: _____ ZIP: _____

Phone number: _____ Fax number: _____

E-mail: _____

Nursing license number: _____

(ANCC requires a unique identifier for each learner.)

1. **According to Shelley Cohen, RN, MS, CEN, what can be argued about the current image of the nursing profession?**
   a. It is much better than it was in 1975
   b. It has not changed
   c. Nurses are always looked down upon
   d. Many nurses do not take pride in their profession

2. **Which part of a nurse's physical image is usually the first thing that affects public perception?**
   a. Communication skills
   b. Time management skills
   c. Sense of humor
   d. Appearance

3. **According to the national survey, which of the following was NOT a suggestion given by respondents on how nurses can improve their image?**
   a. Smile, speak in a clear pleasant voice
   b. Communicate with our patients
   c. Avoid eye contact to make patients more comfortable
   d. Speak to patients and families in a caring manner

4. According to Karen L. Tomajan, MS, RN, BC, CNAA, CRRN, the public image of nursing is important because it affects:

   a. The care nurses provide to patients

   b. Recruitment into the profession

   c. Advances in medical science

   d. Relationships between nursing leaders

5. Which of the following nursing images is LEAST familiar to the public?

   a. Handmaiden

   b. Angel of mercy

   c. Naughty nurse

   d. Research-conducting professional

6. Which of the following initiatives aims to promote a more accurate public image of nursing?

   a. Nurses of America project

   b. National Patient Safety Goals

   c. Interdisciplinary Nursing Quality Research Initiative

   d. Betty Irene Moore Nursing Initiative

7. Which of the following is an example of how power is connected to image?

   a. When a nurse is rewarded for going above expectations

   b. When a nurse tolerates an unacceptable situation and results in feeling powerless

   c. When a nurse is disrespectful to a patient

   d. When staffing levels are adequate

8. How does nursing autonomy contribute to professionalism?

   a. Autonomy requires nurses to have a strong sense of self

   b. Autonomy requires nurses to be intelligent

   c. Autonomy requires nurses to be open-minded

   d. Autonomy requires nurses to create strong work relationships

9. Which of the following is a reason why people resist culture change?

   a. Overdeveloped critical-thinking skills

   b. Independence

   c. Respect for colleagues

   d. Apathy

10. **Which of following strategies should be avoided when aiming to secure buy-in for culture change?**
    a. Implementing changes that cannot affect culture
    b. Identifying the changes needed to enhance professional culture
    c. Defining the positives and negatives of your current nursing culture
    d. Keeping a log of all the changes made in nursing for the year, and communicating them to your nurses

11. **Which of the following is a reason why nurses avoid communicating?**
    a. Fear of putting their patients' care in jeopardy
    b. Fear of improving relationships
    c. Fear of being understood
    d. Fear of being fired

12. **When using the DESC communication model, one must _____.**
    a. Say what the nurse should have done
    b. Explain the effect of the behavior
    c. Continue on, despite their frustrations
    d. Describe their frustrations

13. **Which of the following is a characteristic of professional communication?**
    a. Working cooperatively, despite feelings of dislike
    b. Providing criticism, even if in public places
    c. Being respectful of the coworkers you like
    d. Participating in gossip

14. **Which of the following Forces of Magnetism is related to the nursing image?**
    a. Force 10
    b. Force 12
    c. Force 15
    d. Force 17

15. **What is the role of nursing image in the ANCC Magnet Recognition Program®?**
    a. It is promoted positively
    b. It is promoted negatively
    c. It is promoted with standard patient care practices
    d. It is promoted with the urgent need for nurses worldwide

16. **Which of the following is NOT an easy-to-implement strategy to promote nursing staff?**
    a. Published leadership profiles
    b. Organizational and departmental internal and external Web sites
    c. National media
    d. Newsletters

17. **Which of the following is part of the criteria for judging nursing excellence?**
    a. Sporadic improvements in productivity and patient flow rates
    b. Learning environments that support nurses academically and through continuing education and specialty certification
    c. Standard patient, nurse, and physician satisfaction surveys
    d. Nurses that do not belong to professional organizations

18. **How can managers encourage staff to strive for professional excellence?**
    a. Blogging about negative nursing experiences to teach staff members what they should not do
    b. Focusing on pay increases
    c. Creating bulletin boards displaying nursing research projects conducted at your workplace
    d. Displaying a dashboard in enclosed areas with patient care

19. **Which of the following is NOT a method nurses today use to carry out their ethical responsibilities?**
    a. Obtaining advanced degrees in ethics
    b. Writing books and articles about ethics
    c. Serving on ethics committees
    d. Mimicking ethical practices at other facilities

20. **How do nursing ethics relate to professionalism?**
    a. All nurses can succeed by practicing a strict code of ethics
    b. Some nursing boards have incorporated a code of ethics into the rules of their practice act
    c. Strong ethics guarantee improved patient care
    d. Evidence states nurses practicing strong ethics are more likely to be promoted

21. **How can an ethical image of nursing be promoted?**
    a. By providing values and ethics education to help individuals translate good beliefs into ethical behaviors and responses
    b. By ignoring perceptions related to ethics and integrity
    c. By focusing on large changes
    d. By hiring and promoting people that look like they are ethical

22. Media portrayals of nursing usually contain:

    a. Physician-centric care

    b. Multitudes of unidentified nurses

    c. Nurses performing highly skilled tasks

    d. Discussion of nursing patient care issues

23. The Center for Nursing Advocacy issues an award for the 10 best and 10 worst media depictions of the year. The award is called:

    a. The golden stethoscope award

    b. The golden nurse award

    c. The golden lamp award

    d. The image of nursing award

24. One of the ways managers can encourage staff to focus on presenting a positive image of nursing is to promote positive interaction at all levels of the organization by:

    a. Hiring more nursing assistants

    b. Facilitating positive physician relationships and intervening when negative encounters occur

    c. Holding regular office hours

    d. Starting a journal club to examine evidence-based practice articles

25. In 2008, a nurse occupies the position of Commissioner of Public Health for which state?

    a. Massachusetts

    b. New York

    c. North Carolina

    d. Tennessee

26. One of the ways nursing faculty can shape nursing students' image of nursing is by:

    a. Focusing on superficial accoutrements like clothing and personal adornments

    b. Assessing the relevancy of professionalism's meanings and its implications within the wider cultural context

    c. Focusing only on disease processes, treatments, procedures, and tasks

    d. Teaching to the exam

CONTINUING EDUCATION EVALUATION

Name: _____

Title: _____

Facility name: _____

Address: _____

Address: _____

City: _____ State: _____ ZIP: _____

Phone number: _____ Fax number: _____

E-mail: _____

Nursing license number: _____

(ANCC requires a unique identifier for each learner.)

Date completed: _____

1. **This activity met the learning objectives stated:**
    ❏ Strongly Agree   ❏ Agree   ❏ Disagree   ❏ Strongly Disagree

2. **Objectives were related to the overall purpose/goal of the activity:**
    ❏ Strongly Agree   ❏ Agree   ❏ Disagree   ❏ Strongly Disagree

3. **This activity was related to my continuing education needs:**
    ❏ Strongly Agree   ❏ Agree   ❏ Disagree   ❏ Strongly Disagree

4. **The exam for the activity was an accurate test of the knowledge gained:**
    ❏ Strongly Agree   ❏ Agree   ❏ Disagree   ❏ Strongly Disagree

5. **The activity avoided commercial bias or influence:**
    ❏ Strongly Agree   ❏ Agree   ❏ Disagree   ❏ Strongly Disagree

6. **This activity met my expectations:**
    ❏ Strongly Agree   ❏ Agree   ❏ Disagree   ❏ Strongly Disagree

7. **Will this activity enhance your professional practice?**
    ❏ Yes   ❏ No

8. The format was an appropriate method for delivery of the content for this activity:

    ❏ Strongly Agree   ❏ Agree   ❏ Disagree   ❏ Strongly Disagree

9. If you have any comments on this activity please note them here:

_____

_____

_____

_____

_____

_____

_____

10. How much time did it take for you to complete this activity?

_____

_____

Thank you for completing this evaluation of our continuing education activity!

Return completed form to:

HCPro, Inc. • Attn: Continuing Education Manager • 75 Sylvan Street, Suite A-101, Danvers, MA 01923 • Tel 877/727-1728 • Fax 781/639-2982